TESTIMONIALS FROM DR. ROSEMAN'S PATIENTS

"When you first told me about the diet, I thought you were crazy, but now that I have lost forty-two pounds, I feel very differently."

—Aspasia Nikolaou, Ph.D.

"'No hope, Doctor. I can't lose weight.' He had heard that before. So he gave me his book, *The Addictocarb Diet*, and proved me wrong. In the first five weeks I lost fifteen pounds. This creative, informative, and concise approach to weight loss is amazing. And it works!"

—Richard Jeske, Ph.D.

"This diet is brilliant in its simplicity and ability to adapt in the busy, stress-filled western lifestyle. Unlike other diet regimens, the recommendations are simple, pragmatic, and easy to remember . . . During the recent illness and unexpected passing of my brother, I was able to continue to apply the Addictocarb principles to assure I was making healthy food choices during this stressful time in my life."

—Corinne Gamper

"The Addictocarb Diet gets results. It is not a quick fix but rather a way to eat healthy for the long-term while losing weight that stays off. The secret to its success is that you do not feel deprived due to the alternatives Dr. Roseman provides to bread, pasta, and white potatoes. They are completely satisfying."

—Jennifer Grubman Rothenberg, President of Innovative Philanthropy, LLC

"It's been three months since I started the Addictocarb Diet. My jeans are looser and the visceral fat that appeared at menopause, and with which I have been trying to make peace, is slowly melting away."

—Meryl Weiss

"Just had the cauliflower pizza—*wow*! Amazing recipe, thanks so much!"

—Andrew Heller

"Your diet is amazing. I'm so happy that other people are going to be able to take control over their eating the way I have."

—Schele Williams

THE
ADDICTOCARB
DIET

THE
ADDICTOCARB
DIET

AVOID THE 9 HIGHLY ADDICTIVE CARBS
WHILE EATING ANYTHING
ELSE YOU WANT

BRUCE ROSEMAN, M.D.

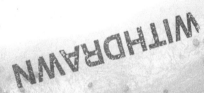

BenBella Books, Inc.
Dallas, Texas

This book is for informational purposes only. It is not intended to serve as a substitute for professional medical advice. The author and publisher specifically disclaim any and all liability arising directly or indirectly from the use of any information contained in this book. A health care professional should be consulted regarding your specific medical situation. Any product mentioned in this book does not imply endorsement of that product by the author or publisher.

BenBella

BenBella Books, Inc.
10300 N. Central Expressway
Suite #530
Dallas, TX 75231
www.benbellabooks.com
Send feedback to feedback@benbellabooks.com

Printed in the United States of America
10 9 8 7 6 5 4 3 2 1

Library of Congress Cataloging-in-Publication Data
Roseman, Bruce.
    The addictocarb diet: avoid the 9 highly addictive carbs while eating anything else you want / by Bruce Roseman, M.D.
        pages cm
    Includes bibliographical references and index.
    ISBN 978-1-941631-08-9 (hardback) — ISBN 978-1-941631-09-6 (electronic)
1. Reducing diets. 2. Low-carbohydrate diet. 3. Reducing diets—Recipes.
4. Low-carbohydrate diet—Recipes. 5. Weight loss. I. Title.
    RM222.2.R6474 2015
    613.2'833—dc23

                                                                2014049122

Editing by Heather Butterfield
    and Vy Tran
Copyediting by James Fraleigh
Proofreading by Jenny Bridges
    and Michael Fedison
Indexing by Debra Bowman
Cover design by Ty Nowicki

Jacket design by Sarah Dombrowsky
Text design by Publishers' Design and
    Production Services, Inc.
Text composition by Integra Software
    Services Pvt. Ltd.
Printed by Lake Book Manufacturing

Distributed by Perseus Distribution
www.perseusdistribution.com

To place orders through Perseus Distribution:
Tel: (800) 343-4499
Fax: (800) 351-5073
E-mail: orderentry@perseusbooks.com

Significant discounts for bulk sales are available. Please contact Glenn Yeffeth at glenn@benbellabooks.com or (214) 750-3628.

*This book is dedicated to my wife, Ellen,
and my sons, Joshua and Aaron, because,
after all, they are everything.*

Contents

Part Four: Eating for Your Health

Part Five: The Addictocarb Diet Recipes and Menus

Appendices

Acknowledgments

The list of acknowledgments is long, but I could never have written this book without the expert editing, ideas, and support of my best friend, Larry Lynn. Ken Rosenberg, who wrote the terrific Foreword, has been a source of constant support as well as insight into addiction. Marcia Amsterdam kept me calm during the entire process, just as she did for my first book. My editor, Heather Butterfield, was really able to visualize the big picture as well as the minutiae and as a result tremendously improved the book. My agent, Matthew Carlini, for his unfaltering belief in the book and getting me not only a good publisher (BenBella) but also the right publisher. To Carla Levy, a long-standing patient of mine, a former executive editor at Condé Nast, who was in the office one day and just said, "Hey, if you want, I could take a look at it and give you some advice." I can only say, "Whew!" and, "Thank you, thank you, thank you!" She improved the book immeasurably. My nurses past and present, Donna, Mandie, and Nicole, for being sounding boards and food tasters. Finally, to all my patients, for their efforts in helping me sculpt this diet over the years by offering suggestions and providing me with invaluable feedback, support, and of course recipes.

Foreword

It's been said that you are what you eat. In fact, according to the emerging science of addiction, *you are a prisoner of what you eat.* Many hedonic (or pleasure-inducing) foods, such as carbohydrates, are known to hijack the reward and reason centers in the brain and create new cellular memories, which then direct and control your future food choices. So at lunch we are prisoners of breakfast. In middle age we are prisoners of our childhood habits. In old age we are infirm with diseases arising from a lifetime of altered brain and body receptors.

And here's an interesting fact: The consequences of our flawed eating habits don't stop at death! New data in the field of epigenetics shows that our eating habits alter our DNA and affect the eating habits of our offspring and possibly succeeding generations. So not only are *you* what you eat but *your grandchildren also are what you eat!*

How is this all possible? Blame evolution, which has provided us with a flexible brain and body that can quickly adapt to new dietary conditions regardless of whether those conditions are good for us. This is the crux of how addictions take hold—the fast-acting, less-discriminating reward and decision systems prevail over slower, more thoughtful, discriminating decision processes. Feeding rats addictive carbohydrates will result in successive generations of those animals with altered DNA that are prepared for this new dietary environment. The rats' babies will have new, if unhealthy, eating habits to enable them to eat in the carb-laden environment of their grandparents. This radical new idea in genetics teaches us that our genes can change quickly to anticipate new climates.

There are two things evolution didn't count on. One, evolution needs us to live just long enough to bear children and has no concern with the quality or length of lives. Therefore, our brains may modify our eating habits with little regard for our long-term health and happiness. Second, evolution didn't count on refrigerators, processed food, and manipulative "food science" manufacturers who trick our brains into addictive eating cycles that are bad for us. In sum, our body and brain, and our genes and gene modulators, have been hoodwinked by shrewd marketers who have ushered us into an addictive relationship with cheap, unhealthy foods.

Dr. Bruce Roseman has a way to stop, fight back, and win! His diet system is easy, fun, and delicious. I know because I've been a guinea pig for his recipes. In plain language, he harnesses the new findings in addiction neuroscience and packages them into a manageable plan to make them accessible for everyone. It will motivate you to mount an offensive on addictive food habits.

Dr. Roseman's diet system is a start for breaking out of the addictive cycle. He puts the food addict on the right path. His wisdom and personal testimonies are inspirational. Read this book and begin on a path of health and mindful eating, with knowledge that may change your life forever.

—Kenneth Paul Rosenberg, M.D.
New York, New York

Kenneth Paul Rosenberg, M.D., is an acclaimed addiction specialist and filmmaker. He is an editor of the landmark textbook on addiction *Behavioral Addictions: Criteria, Evidence, and Treatment.* He is a board-certified addiction psychiatrist and a clinical associate professor of psychiatry at the

New York-Presbyterian/Weill Cornell Medical Center and has been recognized in the Best Doctors in America® database and in *New York Magazine*'s Best Doctors list of top addiction psychiatrists. Dr. Rosenberg is the founder and director of Upper East Health Behavioral Medicine in Manhattan, a psychiatric practice that provides treatment for individuals and families recovering from chemical and behavioral addictions.

INTRODUCTION:
MY STORY

I was one of millions of people hooked on what I call "Addictocarbs." They killed my father and are killing millions more. This book is my story and my solution. My solution is based not just on personal anecdotes or salvation but on thousands of pages of investigation, clinical observation, and the latest neuroscience research into the global obesity epidemic.

Hello, my name is Bruce and I am an addict—a food addict, that is. I freely admit it. If it were up to me, I would get up in the morning and eat nonstop all day. I would keep a refrigerator next to my bed and raid it at least twice a night. Any spare moments I had I would spend shopping for, cooking, and consuming food. I even love to photograph food. This is how I lived most of my life and why I was always fat. I was a fat kid and a fat adult. A number of years ago I finally had to pay for my lifetime of culinary transgressions when I was diagnosed with diabetes.

I decided I was going to beat diabetes. But *how* was I going to do it? I had already been on virtually every diet over the last fifty years, including all the usual suspects—Atkins, Pritikin, Stillman, Scarsdale, and Weight Watchers. I had been on all-meat diets, the cabbage soup diet, low-carb diets, ultra low-carb diets, high-protein diets, and vegetarian diets. I had lost seventy pounds twice, and each time, as soon as I had lost the weight, I started on a new diet—the "gaining your weight back diet"—and methodically put it back on. I knew that I could *lose* weight on diets; unfortunately, I also knew that I would eventually gain the weight back.

If I was going to beat diabetes, this time had to be different.

You're probably thinking that I live a sedentary lifestyle and that if I got off my behind and exercised more, I would be able to maintain my weight. Wrong! I ran so much for so many years—five to seven miles a day, seven days a week—that I literally wore out the metatarsophalangeal joints in my big toes. I walk with pain even now because of my past obsession with running. When I could no longer run, in desperation I switched to swimming. I have been swimming six to seven days a week for about fifteen years, and at one point I even swam three hours a day. Lack of exercise is not my problem.

Just to end the suspense, let me say that I lost about sixty pounds starting about ten years ago and I have kept it off ever since. It has been easier than ever before. I have never gone this long a period of time being thin. As the weight fell off and I stayed thin, patients began asking me how I did it. I told them, and soon many of my patients were doing it, too.

As I lost weight, my need to experiment and track data came out and I started making charts, keeping a diary, and putting everything in spreadsheets. Soon I had data detailing my blood sugar readings up to ten times per day, at all hours, and after every single type of food that I ate. I weighed myself constantly. I jotted down my observations, not only on everything I ate but also how I felt and how it affected my weight. I know that this is not normal; but then, I was a guy who had previously gained and lost seventy pounds twice. Is *that* normal?

I had obsessively attacked and solved serious medical problems before and had been successful. For instance, when a host of professionals told me and my wife that our son had a pan-developmental disorder and might never learn to read,

I went into high gear. I invented a method to teach my son to read, detailed in my previous book, *A Kid Just Like Me*. It was a very difficult time, but I did it. My son, whom the experts predicted would never read, graduated from the illustrious Bronx High School of Science and Brandeis University. Children across the United States have benefited from my method, so tackling this health issue was not virgin territory to me. I had plastered the house with diagrams and spreadsheets and observations before, and it had worked. I took inspiration from that, and I was ready to do it again.

This time, though, my life was on the line, and I could not help but think of the pain of losing my father when he was fifty-two and I was twenty-one. I did not want that to happen to my sons, now twenty-one and twenty-five, so once again I became obsessed with solving a complicated, serious, multifactorial medical problem.

Solving a problem like this was not really a stretch from what I do for a living. Over the years I had become a "go-to" doctor for patients who had particularly difficult and complicated medical problems. It has given me a fully satisfying life, helping people who thought they could not really be helped. Now I had become one of those people.

I had always assumed that there was no helping me and my food addiction. Like my wife always said, "You've got the pig gene, and there is not much you can do about it." I had always thought she was right. It turns out she *was* right—but she was also wrong.

She was right because, as she so eloquently put it, the "pig gene" is inherited. In fact, there is a gene referred to as D2 or DRD2 that is associated with a variety of addictive behaviors. Though I have never been tested for DRD2, I certainly had inherited overweight tendencies from others in my family who were very fat. My grandparents on my father's side and my uncles and aunts all flirted with 300 pounds. My own father fought the battle of the bulge gallantly for most of his life and was somewhat successful; but, like me, he was always up and down with his weight. He died a young man, and while I firmly believe that today's medical interventions could have prolonged his life, I also believe that the basis for his heart disease was his yo-yoing weight.

One of my favorite patients of all time was a psychologist whom I will refer to as Dr. Q. I learned a lot from her because every time she came in, she would critique my bedside manner. I might have found that hard to take from a lot of people, but not her. First, she was a lot older than me and quite accomplished. Second, she was kind. Third, every time she spoke, I learned something from her. Over many years her critiques of my style of treating her significantly improved my patient interactions, and for that I owe her a debt of gratitude.

I loved talking to Dr. Q about anything under the sun because she was brilliant and insightful. She was also fat—morbidly obese fat. And periodically she used to get thin—anorexic thin. She used to go on medically supervised fasts, consuming a powder drink that a local hospital program provided, which would cause her to lose a tremendous amount of weight. Then she would just as methodically gain it all back.

I had seen it all before. As a young resident doctor, I had worked with one of the very first powder diets at Hahnemann University Hospital in Philadelphia. I knew that it worked. We gave patients the powder, which they made into shakes and drank exclusively in lieu of meals. It worked. They lost weight; unfortunately, they always ended up gaining the weight back.

Dr. Q and I used to talk endlessly about her weight loss and why she could not keep the weight off. If I had to be honest, we were really talking about *our* weight problem. She used to point out that the problem with an eating addiction is special. With most addictions you can only beat them if you completely refrain from the addictive behavior. Take alcohol, for example. If you are an alcoholic, you can only beat it if you accept your addiction and commit to yourself that you will never have another drink. But Dr. Q used to tell me, "Bruce, I have an addiction. I accept that and I can go for a few months on the powder shakes and not eat, but eventually a person has to eat. It is just part of the human condition. And so restarts the addiction once again." She was, of course, right; but as I know now, she was also wrong.

Every week I would go to Zabar's and Fairway Market, two famous food emporiums in Manhattan, and spend countless hours shopping. My wife referred to them as food museums. The smells were intoxicating. Touching the food was intoxicating. Carrying the food home and unpacking it was intoxicating. It was all intoxicating, and I loved it. I was an addict. Addicts love being intoxicated. I was also fat, really fat. I did not love being really fat.

After reading Rose Levy Beranbaum's epic cookbook, *The Cake Bible*, I baked a cake a day, most days, for months. On the days that I was not baking, I was at the stores seeking out various ingredients. I could not possibly eat all the cakes, so I gave most of the cakes away, eating only part of each one. I became a really adept baker. The experience was exhilarating. I gained thirty-five pounds from that endeavor, and I was already considerably overweight.

Once the food networks started on cable TV, I watched them incessantly. My family thought it was funny. I just loved it and figured, no problem, I am just *watching*, not eating. Unfortunately, watching the shows made me hungry, so I ate. I got fatter, and I was fat to begin with.

The day came when I finally had to face the harsh reality that I was eating myself to death—I was diagnosed with diabetes. I went on medication—lots of medication. At first it was just pills and then it progressed to injections. I hated it. I hated being fat and I hated having diabetes and I hated all the medications and the injections. I had to do something about it and I knew it.

The first step was acceptance. I needed to accept the fact that food was my addiction. My wife, who is not a food addict, could get up in the morning and eat six Oreos for breakfast. She did this for years. She never ate five or seven or nine or any other number, just six. That was her breakfast. She stayed thin.

I could never eat *just* six Oreos. I could not even comprehend such a thing. I would eat the whole bag and then open another bag. That is because I am an addict. I would feel the exact same way after eating my first Oreo as I would after eating three full bags of Oreos. I would want another one. I would need another one. I would crave another one. That is how addicts feel after every fix. They want another one. Oh sure, they may not need a fix every hour, but they know it is only a matter of time until they need the next fix. It is only now, with recent addiction research, that we can look at scans of people's brains when they are eating certain foods and see that, in fact, *exactly* the same thing occurs in addicts' brains under the influence of drugs and alcohol.

But more on this later. I was an addict. How was I going to cure my addiction?

I had realized through my constant dieting over the years that there was a point after I started a diet where the cravings lessened. I calculated that there were a number of humps. There was one at about three days, another at about two weeks, and again at about three months. Both times that I lost seventy pounds, it took me about nine months. At that point things were better, but I still had cravings. It struck me that this was much the same pattern you saw when extinguishing any behavior.

I knew I could go on a diet and it would take me a few days to calm down the cravings, and then my body would challenge me with food cravings at about two weeks, and again periodically. That, I reasoned, was because, just like a crying baby or Pavlov's dogs, it was about a habit, a craving—an addiction. You can break the addiction, but the addiction will challenge you again and again.

So, I needed to come up with ways to conquer my addiction and to deal with the inevitable cravings that would resurface in due course.

I realize now that in spite of losing all of that weight, I never really lost my cravings. That was because I was still an addict. I was finding out what Dr. Q had told me about so many years ago: Eventually, you have to go back to eating. And that is just like an alcoholic going back to drinking; it just won't work. However, you *can* go back to eating without setting off addictive behaviors or at the very least with the cravings significantly diminished. I knew that for me the key was carbohydrates.

All the diets I tried over the years had one thing in common: They worked, but I would eventually start to gain my weight back. When I went on the Stillman and Atkins diets, they severely limited carbs, and I lost weight, but I was miserable without my carbs. When I went off those diets I started eating again, trying to watch my diet to keep the weight off by minding my calories and carbs intake, but eventually the cravings got the best of me. I would try to have just a baked potato without the sour cream or butter. I would try to have just one piece of bread with my eggs. I even tried very thinly sliced bread, which had less than half the calories, but still, sooner or later, it would escalate and I would once again be fat. The cravings kept getting the best of me until a number of years ago when I began seeing studies on addiction research. Those studies, my own personal experience, and what I have learned through treating my patients have shaped my new diet.

I call it the Addictocarb Diet. Since starting it, I have lost weight and stayed thin. Over the years, I have recommended it to almost a thousand patients who have also benefited from it. I could never have come to all of these conclusions without my trusty patients, who have helped me shape this diet into what it is today. The Addictocarb Diet, fully detailed in this book, will do for you what it has done for my patients and me.

PART ONE:

How Does Food Addiction Affect You?

CHAPTER 1

The Diet Overview: An Easy Guide to Addictocarbs

Before we delve into the specific steps of the diet, I want to explain a few things. Addictocarbs are foods that work like narcotics on the addiction centers of the brain. Bread, potatoes, alcohol, and cocaine are all addictive substances. They all stimulate the addiction centers of the brain similarly, and they need to be treated similarly. By that I mean what every single addiction treatment program, whether it's Alcoholics Anonymous or a celebrity substance-abuse center, has figured out: You must totally give up the addictive substances. As a result, going through the three steps of this diet is similar to breaking any other addiction. Step 1, shaking the addiction, will be like going through withdrawal. Step 2 will be just like going through rehab, and Step 3 will be about learning ways to live with your addiction.

> What happens when you eat an Addictocarb? The same exact thing that happens when you use any addictive substance. You want more. Just like cocaine, heroin, or alcohol. You just want more and more, and it leads to a bottomless pit with dire consequences.

For a diet to be successful, it needs to not only to treat addiction but also to be palatable, healthy, and sustainable.

The Addictocarb Diet does this in ways that no other diet has in the past. It cures the addiction by identifying and eliminating the most addictive and lethal carbohydrates and by promoting fruits, which low-carb diets like South Beach and Atkins restrict. This diet also offers a wide variety of "Addictocarb Alternatives" and "Addictocarb Accommodations," tasty, healthy dishes that help you avoid the most addictive carbs over the long term. I will point out many reasons that fruits, those powerhouses of antioxidants, and the various Addictocarb Alternatives are good for you, are *not* addictive, and do not raise blood sugar significantly; just as important, they are tasty, and offer dietary variety. While a diet of Brussels sprouts, broccoli, and spinach would work just as well as the Addictocarb Diet, who is likely to stay on it? Why *would* you, if you could get the same results by eating palatable fruits and the various Addictocarb Alternatives, like Dreamfields® pasta and kasha, and the Addictocarb Accommodations, like brown rice and whole wheat pasta, that I will present? They will help you conquer addiction yet still be palatable, healthy, and sustainable. **The bottom line with the Addictocarb Diet is that you can lose your cravings by dealing with your food addiction, you can lose weight, you can sustain that weight loss, and you can conquer diabetes as well as many other diseases.**

The *first* thing you will need to do is to accept that *if* you are overweight, then you have food addiction issues. Perhaps you were just born that way, or perhaps it's something you acquired later in life when circumstances changed. Nevertheless, as a food addict, you get food cravings that lead to addictive behavior, which is part of an addiction syndrome. You need to break the cycle.

Once you *accept* your addiction, you can begin to deal with the problem. As with all addictions, when you try to give them up you go into withdrawal; but with this diet you still get to take in lots of carbs, so the pain of withdrawal is muted.

You will learn that not all carbs are created equal, and you will come to understand the concept of Addictocarbs: carbs that cause intense cravings by stimulating the addiction center of the brain. The Addictocarbs are bread, potatoes, pasta, flour, rice, sugar, high fructose corn syrup, fruit juice, and soda.

> The Addictocarbs are *bread, potatoes, pasta, flour, rice, sugar, high fructose corn syrup, fruit juice, and soda.* The reason I have chosen these nine *specifically* is because I have found in treating my many patients over the years that it is *these* foods and ingredients that have presented them with the greatest addiction challenges.

I have chosen these nine Addictocarbs *specifically* because I have found, over years of treating many, many patients, that *these* foods and ingredients have presented them with the greatest addiction challenges. Also, a quick look at US Department of Agriculture data[1] reveals that consumption of these particular things has increased, paralleling the obesity epidemic in the United States—especially high fructose corn syrup, which was unheard of until forty years ago. You will learn how to beat the addiction to these foods by employing the Shake and, later, Addictocarb Alternatives and Addictocarb Accommodations. You will go through these three steps.

STEP 1: SHAKING THE ADDICTION.

Step 1 lasts for three days. You break your Addictocarb addiction here by consuming nothing but high-calorie, high-carb Shakes. These Addictocarb-free Shakes are what would be referred to in your gym or nutrition store as a health shake. The Shake is my version of it. It contains milk (cow, soy, or almond), fruits, and a flavoring powder. While it is high in carbs and calories, it does not contain any Addictocarbs. The point is to wean you off Addictocarbs, not all carbs. During this time, you *will* experience withdrawal symptoms or cravings, just like you would at the beginning of any diet. They will be most intense in the first few days, but you will be shocked how quickly they fade away because of the Shakes.

Can you put up with cravings for a few days? I believe you can with these high-calorie, high-carb Shakes.

After the first three days, you will have drastically reduced your cravings, just like an addict going through withdrawal. You will feel cleansed and triumphant. By the way, you will also lose weight. But remember, while the point of this diet is to lose weight, it is mostly about staying thin once you have taken it off. Understanding how easy it is to give up Addictocarbs is an important step in laying the groundwork for a thin and healthy life.

STEP 2: ADDICTOCARB REHAB

Step 2 lasts for two weeks. You cannot eat Addictocarbs during this time—no bread, potatoes, pasta, flour, rice, sugar, high fructose corn syrup, fruit juice, or soda. On the other hand, there are things you *can* eat, such as fruits, salads, vegetables, cheese, nuts, beans, and proteins such as meat, chicken, fish, and tofu. I will also provide some Addictocarb Alternatives—foods that mimic Addictocarbs but are tasty, healthy, and *non*-addictive—such as Dreamfields pasta for pasta and kasha for rice. (Many of these dos and don'ts of food are listed in convenient chart form in Appendix B.)

The challenge of Addictocarb rehab varies for each individual, depending on how much Addictocarb food one is accustomed to eating. For example, if you are like most people in America and virtually all of my patients, then you probably eat quite a lot of Addictocarbs. For those of you who are having the most difficult time, you can partake of some of the provided Addictocarb Alternatives for bread, pasta, and potatoes. The important thing to remember is that we are setting the stage for a future healthier life. So while you might lose more weight staying off the Addictocarb Alternatives, you will still lose weight even with them.

STEP 3: STAYING THIN FOR LIFE

Step 3 lasts for as long as you want it to. It will set the stage for the rest of your life. In addition to the Addictocarb Alternatives from Step 2 for bread, pasta, and potatoes, I introduce some fascinating Addictocarb Alternatives for rice and snacks. Also, for those of you who are feeling that you either do not want to give up rice, pasta, and flour, or cannot at this point, I present the concept of Addictocarb *Accommodations*, things like brown rice and whole wheat spaghetti. If you prefer to employ these, you might not lose as much weight or lose it as quickly, but you will still lose weight successfully and keep it off.

You will have to decide here which Addictocarbs you will banish from your diet completely and which you will allow on a limited basis. The important thing is that you will be able to make these decisions without the pull of addiction.

Let's face it. If you want to stay thin, you will have to give up something; at the most basic level, either bread or potatoes, preferably both. Does this mean that for the rest of your life you will never be able to eat another potato or a piece of bread? I would like to say yes, but the reality of that happening is unlikely. I will explain to you how to deal with the occasional transgression, planned and unplanned, and even how to deal with falling off the wagon. I will discuss some of my personal recipes and talk about others'. I will mention some foods that have worked for me and for my patients. I will describe some typical meals that have been successful for me and my patients over the years.

You will be surprised at how different you will become. Unlike other diets where you enter maintenance with dread because you know in your heart the cravings will return, you will be exhilarated by how powerful you feel having conquered your addiction. In the chapter on Addictocarb bonus health benefits, I will talk about diabetes, because I have it and because it is an out-of-control epidemic in this country and around the world. I will discuss how the Addictocarb Diet, contrary to accepted medical wisdom—which says you should *not* eat a lot of carbs—has transformed my diabetes and helped my diabetic patients. I will also talk about it because according to the American Diabetes Association's data from the 2014 *National Diabetes Statistics Report,* there are approximately 100 million diabetics and prediabetics in this country,[2] and it is the most significant medical issue confronting the American population today. Last, at the end of this book you'll find answers to frequently asked questions and an appendix with helpful material including a complete list of what you can and can't eat during the various stages of the diet.

Now, it is almost time to get started losing some weight and staying thin. But before we do, I would like to explain some things about food addiction.

CHAPTER 2

Looking at Food as an Addictive Substance

THE SCIENCE OF FOOD ADDICTION

According to the American Society of Addiction Medicine, "Addiction is characterized by inability to consistently abstain, impairment in behavioral control, craving, diminished recognition of significant problems with one's behaviors and interpersonal relationships, and a dysfunctional emption response. Like other chronic diseases, addiction often involves cycles of relapse and remission. Without treatment or engagement in recovery activities, addiction is progressive and can result in disability or premature death."[1]

You can evaluate a heroin addict or an alcoholic and realize that the person is in trouble. What is more difficult is looking at a successful fifty-year-old doctor who is fifty pounds overweight and recognizing that he, too, is an addict and in deep trouble. He might not fit the picture of an addict, but he is. Like heroin addiction, the doctor's addiction will cause significant medical problems that are less obvious but are just as lethal, including high blood pressure, stroke, heart disease, diabetes, higher incidences of certain cancers, and the list goes on.

I was that doctor. I was an addict, even though I did not think of myself as one. You, reading this book to lose weight, might not consider yourself an addict, but you have likely engaged in addictive behaviors. Perhaps you became a food addict because you were genetically or prenatally predisposed, or you acquired terrible eating habits growing up; often the cause is rooted in the stresses of life we all endure. Nevertheless, all these paths lead to the same destination—food addiction. Otherwise, you would probably be thin. Any time you get a craving to buy potato chips, you are exhibiting addictive behavior. Just *looking* at the potato chips will stimulate the addictive center of the brain. Unbelievable though it may sound, medicine can now prove this with brain scans. Dr. David S. Ludwig, the director of the Obesity Prevention Center at Boston Children's Hospital, did brain scans in men, giving them the foods and ingredients that I call Addictocarbs, and "the scans showed intense activation in brain regions involved in addictive behavior."[2] Even for a doctor familiar with fast-moving medical advances this is a staggering finding, but it does not end there. There is further support for the food addiction model in the medical literature. An article in *The Archives of General Psychiatry* explains that the addiction center of the brain lights up the same way whether it's responding to heroin or certain foods.[3] Yet another article from the *American Journal of Clinical Nutrition* sums it up beautifully and succinctly when it states that "some foods are more powerful than others at stimulating the addictive areas of the brain."[4]

In short, excellent medical studies done by top researchers at major medical institutions are showing up at an increasing rate, reinforcing and proving what many world-class medical addiction specialists like Dr. Kenneth Paul Rosenberg have been saying for years. In his recently published landmark medical textbook, *Behavioral Addictions*,[5] the chapter on food

addiction alone has eleven full pages of references—
something that would have been unimaginable just a few
short years ago. What is clear is that the scientific community has accepted that certain foods stimulate the addiction
center of the brain, and it is these addictive food cravings that
promote obesity.

Medicine only recently accepted food addiction as a real
condition when, in May 2014, the American Psychiatric Association finally included food addiction in the fifth edition of
its psychiatric "bible," the *Diagnostic and Statistical Manual
of Mental Disorders*, classifying it under "Feeding and Eating
Disorders."[6] Many clinicians, myself included, believe it should
have been placed under "Substance-Related and Addictive
Disorders," but it nevertheless shows real progress for food
addiction gaining acceptance. The point is that food addiction
is now considered scientific fact by the medical establishment.

Food addiction is even showing up in features in popular
magazines, on TV shows, and in classrooms. In a 2011 *Time*
article, neuroscience journalist Maia Szalavitz asks the question, "Is Häagen-Dazs ice cream as addictive as heroin? Or,
put another way, is heroin as addictive as Häagen-Dazs?"[7]
Dr. Nora Volkow, a nationally recognized authority who has
spent a lifetime studying addiction and who is the director
of the National Institute on Drug Abuse, has said repeatedly on *60 Minutes*[8] and in her lectures[9] that overeating is
an addiction.

Here is the real question: Is a person who eats things
like bread and potatoes, and as a result is twenty-five pounds
overweight, an addict? To most of the researchers the answer
to that question would technically be no, even though most
authorities would agree that the brain center for addiction
is stimulated as it would be by drugs. To me, however, the
answer is a resounding yes. That is because I have a unique
perspective. As a family doctor, I get to see the havoc that
being overweight wreaks on patients' lives. I see the toll it

takes on families. Every year I see people suffer and even die prematurely because of heart disease or some other malady caused by being overweight. It devastates their families and it breaks my heart.

Alcohol or cocaine abuse is considered an addiction by most because the dire consequences are clear to anyone observing these users' behaviors. We witness the physical deterioration of the addict and how the addiction becomes central to their life. But what about having a few fries or a roll with dinner? When you consider the staggering prevalence of Addictocarb addiction, and the devastating results of that addiction, I think you have to put Addictocarbs up there with heroin, alcohol, and cocaine *combined*.

I believe that the main cause of obesity and type 2 diabetes is Addictocarbs, which can be appreciated by looking at the FDA data on increases in food consumption that parallel the obesity epidemic. Just consider that there are about 70 million prediabetics in the country and another 30 million diagnosed diabetics, while total cocaine and heroin addicts measure fewer than 4 million (though as you can imagine, this number is open to debate). But whatever the real number, it clearly pales in comparison to Addictocarb addiction. In society as a whole, food addiction far outweighs drug and alcohol addiction in its health consequences, and we all pay for this in our taxes, health insurance premiums, and quality of life. If we cut Addictocarbs from the Standard American Diet, we would wipe out most obesity, type 2 diabetes, heart disease, many cancers, and a whole host of other diseases. In fact, just cutting out *one* Addictocarb from our diet would dramatically impact the health of this country.

Overeating and eating many of the wrong foods are symptoms of an addiction, and if you do not accept that fact and treat certain foods like an addiction, you will never be able to *stay* thin. Cycling through diets and weight loss is just like going into substance abuse rehab over and over. But food addiction may be even worse. Dr. Kelly D. Brownell, who coined the term "yo-yo dieting" and has published widely and served on the faculties of the University of Pennsylvania, Yale University, and Duke University, famously discusses the possible metabolic and health consequences of yo-yo dieting. In a study on which he was lead author, "The Effects of Repeated Cycles of Weight Loss and Regain in Rats," his data suggests a specific point: Frequent dieting may make subsequent weight loss more difficult.[10]

But yo-yo dieting isn't the only problem. Even trying to *force* yourself to go on a prolonged diet with surgical interventions will not work because the problem is not the eating; it is the addiction. For example, people who have had stomach stapling or gastric sleeves stop their bulk eating, but the addiction continues unabated. As with any addiction, people find ways around it or even develop alternate addictions, such as cocaine or alcohol.[11]

I have seen it in my practice. It is what addicts do. They will do anything to get their fix. The problem with getting stomach surgery is that people are still allowed to eat what they want, just in smaller quantities. If before your gastric bypass you consumed a hundred M&Ms at a sitting, now you can eat ten an hour for ten hours without discomfort. This is not going to work. It doesn't work for alcohol or heroin, and it won't work for food. The only thing that works is completely giving up the substance being abused.

The first question that comes up is: What are the most addictive foods? The answer to that question is Addictocarbs. The second question is: How do you give them up? The answer to that question is through substituting healthful, appetizing foods for the Addictocarbs. That is what the Addictocarb Diet will do: It will get you to completely give up the addictive substances by replacing them with palatable, nonaddictive alternatives.

So to lose weight and keep it off, you have to be able to completely give up the addictive substances, and you can only do that by controlling your cravings. How can that be done?

HUNGER VERSUS CRAVINGS

Hunger is a biological need and is often associated with physical sensations like contractions of the stomach muscles (growling), or a feeling of stomach emptiness, though it may also involve feelings of light-headedness and weakness. It does not involve a particular food or drink. Cravings, on the other hand, usually do involve particular foods, such as potato chips or Oreos, and are often caused by addiction issues resulting from eating Addictocarbs, or emotional issues, such as depression. Cravings might last for a long time, but eventually you will get over them or just lose interest and crave something else. By contrast, hunger might pass momentarily, but it will come back, or its symptoms will worsen.

It *cannot* be done long term by going on low-carb, high-protein diets like the Atkins Diet because people cannot stay on them for very long, not to mention that they are not very good for you. I was on Atkins, and I lost weight. Unfortunately, I got pretty sick of just eating hamburger patties and lamb chops, and I could never really get rid of my cravings for carbs. As soon as I went off the diet, I just started a new diet—the "gaining your weight back" diet.

It *cannot* be done by going on fasts. Diets that want you to fast are popular, but once again, how long can you stay on a fast? Some recent popular diets recommend intermittent fasting. I suppose this can work, but the cravings will also be intermittent, and that will not work any better than an alcoholic who only drinks on the weekends.

It *cannot* be done by going on a low-glycemic-index diet like South Beach. While these kinds of diets are better than

Atkins and fasting, they cut down but do not cut out the addictive substances, thus allowing, and even facilitating, reemergence of addictive eating. Also, these diets restrict healthful, nonaddictive foods like fruit that can be of great benefit in a permanent weight loss program like the Addictocarb Diet.

Many diets can help you lose weight, and they all work in the short term, but unless you deal with the issue of addiction, they ultimately fail. As I have learned the hard way, after every fad diet comes another diet—the "gaining your weight back" diet. Everyone basically knows this, though some may not want to accept it. When you are finally willing to deal with your food addiction, you will learn to conquer it. Treat being overweight just like any other addiction. Go through the steps of giving up an addiction: detox, rehab, and dealing with your life as an addict.

The only thing that *will* work is a diet that is commonsensical. By this I mean a diet that gets rid of your strongest cravings and yet still allows you to have carbs and enjoy the sensual pleasures of eating. The question that comes up is whether all carbs are created equal. Here, too, data suggests that there are certain carbs, which I refer to as Addictocarbs, that cause more intense cravings. It is the premise of this diet that the absolute worst carbs that cause the most cravings are Addictocarbs: bread, potatoes, pasta, flour, rice, sugar, high fructose corn syrup, fruit juice, and soda. But what about carbs in general?

CARBS, ADDICTOCARBS, AND FOOD ADDICTION

Let's talk about carbs. Some carbs are good, and some carbs are bad. Fruits are good carbs. Vegetables are good carbs. Other carbs, the ones I call Addictocarbs, are bad carbs.

Carbohydrates in general get a bad rap. Dieters think that by eating fewer carbs they will lose weight and keep it off. The truth is that it is hard to live with carbs, but you certainly cannot live without them. Carbs perform vital functions. Some provide the fuel you live on, some are stored by your body to provide energy for later consumption, and others play critical roles in your immune system, fertilization process, blood clotting, and more. But not all carbs are created equal.

Addictocarbs are carbs that cause addictive behaviors. To me, addictive behaviors are those that cause people to eat too much or eat the wrong foods. They cause people to buy certain foods on impulse, or because they smell so good that they are irresistible. French fries are Addictocarbs. So are bread and rolls and cupcakes. Pasta and rice are Addictocarbs. Fruits, while chock full of carbs, are not Addictocarbs. The Addictocarb Alternatives that I give in the book also have lots of carbs, but they are not Addictocarbs. We will discuss what are and are not Addictocarbs when we get into Step 2 of the diet in chapter six.

A FEW SHORT WORDS ABOUT FATS

In all this talk about carbs and Addictocarbs, one question comes up: What about fats? At the beginning of this chapter I talked about how carbs get a bad rap. The same applies to fats. You literally cannot live without them. Fats are required to metabolize vitamins A, D, E, and K. They play a vital role in everything from cushioning your organs against shock to ensuring the efficient functioning of your immune system.

Additionally, no-fat food is often high in sugar. Sugar is an Addictocarb—not the worst Addictocarb, mind you, but an Addictocarb nonetheless. Addictocarbs cause cravings, so I am generally opposed to low-fat foods if they contain lots of sugar. If they don't, they are fine. But you have to check. Many trendy diets over the years have been based on high fats and low carbs. Without commenting on the health consequences of high-fat diets, the very fact that so many high-fat diets exist confirms that you can eat lots of fat and lose weight. Also, all the low-glycemic diets allow fats because the glycemic index of fat is very low.

> The glycemic index is a measure of how quickly a given food is converted to sugar in the gastrointestinal tract, and then how quickly it is absorbed into the bloodstream. It is a general way to gauge whether a food is fattening.

Many years ago I went on the Stillman Diet, which was similar to the Atkins Diet and so many others. I ate bacon, cheese, hamburger patties, and other high-fat foods until it was coming out of my ears, and I still lost weight. Many people lose weight on those diets. My suspicion is that all of those people put the weight back on just as I did.

I do not worry about any food except those that cause cravings, especially Addictocarbs. I personally prefer to eat naturally low-fat foods because I feel better when I do, and I do not think that a lot of fat is good for you, especially for cardiovascular health. But it does not really have a bearing on this diet. *The Addictocarb Diet* makes it simple; it helps you understand which foods, by virtue of their addictive properties, undermine your sincerest efforts to lose weight and keep it off.

I do know three things for sure in terms of weight loss: Addictocarbs are bad for you, fruit is good for you, and fats can go either way. Whether fats cause other issues, such as heart disease, is a totally different matter, worthy of discussion with your doctor and for other books to take up.

MOVING THROUGH LIFE AS A FOOD ADDICT: IT STARTS YOUNG AND GOES DOWNHILL FROM THERE

I love children's birthday parties because I love children. I cannot think of a more fun thing to do than to be in a room full of kids. Yet I am often shocked when I see some parents tussling with their children, attempting to feed birthday cake to their one-year-old baby. The baby turns away from the cake and ice cream as the parent holds the squirming child and gently but forcefully maneuvers the cake into the child's mouth. I marvel at how vigorously these children try to avoid it and how hard the parents have to work to get them to try it. That is, until they get that first taste. Then the addiction begins. They want more, and as soon as they get older they will ask for it. The addiction has taken hold. Like any other addictive substance, party foods seem harmless enough to give to a child, but before you know it they are addicted. I doubt an alcoholic really thinks their first drink will lead to alcoholism or the heroin addict's first dose to addiction. But then the cravings start and BOOM!

I understand that parents think a birthday is a time of celebration, and part of celebration is eating cake. I also know that a one-year-old baby has absolutely no understanding of the concept of birthdays or of celebrating with cake. This is a learned behavior. Just like addiction.

A colleague of mine had a revelation recently at the entrance to a big box store. Some Girl Scouts and their mothers had set up long tables there, laden with the traditional Girl Scout cookies. Thin Mints sat beside Samoas and Tagalongs. My colleague remembered his years of selling the cookies in his office to help his daughter achieve her quota. Then he thought about *The Addictocarb Diet*, which he had read in draft form. He was astonished by his revelation. The cookies amount to a large revenue source for Girl Scouts with a staggering number of boxes of these tasty Addictocarbs finding their way into homes across the nation. Young girls are conditioned to believe that the cookies are part and parcel of the goodness of Girl Scouting itself, when, in fact, they are really bad for you. Just like the birthday cake, Girl Scout cookie sales are another subliminal social mechanism for promoting the consumption of Addictocarbs.

Most people do not think of giving a baby a piece of birthday cake or buying Girl Scout cookies as having anything to do with addiction; but then, most people do not consider themselves addicted when performing some of the simple things in life. For example, Hollywood movies frequently tell girls and women that consuming copious amounts of ice cream is an effective and acceptable way of dealing with sadness.

Most people also do not think of purchasing a few French fries or walking down the cookie aisle at the supermarket as signs of addiction. But you need to put it in context. If, by walking down a supermarket aisle, you feel *compelled* to purchase something that is completely self-destructive, then that is an addictive behavior. It is no different than an alcoholic walking down the same supermarket's beer aisle.

It is easy to see why you would refer to an alcoholic's purchase of beer as an addictive behavior. He may purchase a few six-packs, drink some of them, and get behind the wheel of a car and drive; he may be mean to his family; he may do poorly at his job and maybe even get fired. Not to mention the medical issues that come with alcohol addiction, like liver disease. So it is easy to see how this purchase is an addictive behavior.

But what about the fifty-year-old doctor who peruses the shelves of the same market? He skips the beer aisle because he does not drink; instead, he buys some plain potatoes, which he fully intends to bake and eat without butter or sour cream. He buys a loaf of fresh French bread. He plans to have dinner that night with his family, when he will eat the baked potato with some carrots and spinach and a steak. He may eat too much of the French bread throughout dinner and maybe have a second baked potato. He feels that this is a good meal.

While the doctor thinks pretty well of himself, he does not accept the reality that his "good" meal is one that will lead to high blood pressure, stroke, heart disease, diabetes, and a host of serious medical issues that may cause him to die at a young age—just like his father before him.

The real issue here is whether that doctor has any choice, in the same way that the alcoholic may not have a choice. The alcoholic cannot help himself—he is an addict—but the doctor cannot help himself, either, for he, too, is an addict. The same area of both the doctor's and the alcoholic's brains is stimulated as they walk down their respective aisles. They are both indulging in self-destructive addictive behavior. They are both addicts and they both probably started their addiction at a tender age. While it is easier never to start an addiction, it is never too late to *deal* with an addiction.

CHAPTER 3

Two Myths about Weight Loss

Exercise is a great thing for everyone. I am a huge advocate and I live by what I say. I swim for forty-five minutes every day and, despite the pain resulting from years of running, walk two to three miles per day. Exercise is great for your cardiovascular system, diabetes, muscle tone, and bone density. The idea that exercise leads to weight loss, though, is a fundamental myth of modern medicine. Nevertheless, doctors, nutritionists, and others persist in perpetuating this myth.

One of the main reasons that it took me so long to lose weight and sustain that weight loss is that I bought into the concept of weight loss by exercise. I learned it in medical school, it was reinforced in my residency, and the reading I did on nutrition during my early years in practice simply served to further reinforce that belief.

Looking back on my weight issues over the course of my life, what stands out most clearly is the seventy pounds that I lost *twice*, and my most recent sixty-pound weight loss. The one common thing about all of these time periods is that while I increased my exercise dramatically, I also went on a diet. I *assumed* that increased exercise and dieting both explained how I lost so much weight. I was wrong.

A patient who I had not seen for a while came in to see me recently. I commented that she had lost weight. She looked at me and said, "You know what it is? When I was in about a year ago, you told me to stop worrying about doing so much exercise and just stay away from most Addictocarbs. I am shocked at how well it has worked out. I no longer worry about doing so much exercise, and aside from staying away from some Addictocarbs, I do not really watch my diet much." I smiled and remembered my own struggles with exercise, diet, and weight.

People who perpetuate the myth about exercise and weight loss look at one fact: Supposedly, when you exercise enough to burn off 3,500 calories if you are a man, or 2,700 calories if you are a woman, you should lose a pound of weight. I disagree. Over the years I have seen many, many people come in and tell me that they are burning off calories at the gym and could not understand why they were not losing weight. I even did my own personal weight loss study by exercising 3.5 hours per day for three months, only to find that I did not lose one single ounce. Once I finally figured out that losing weight has nothing to do with exercise, and I explained this to my patients, I was finally able to get people to lose weight by simply changing their diet. It took me a little while longer to understand that while you will lose weight with pretty much any diet, the only way to lose weight and keep it off is to deal with addiction issues. Thus the Addictocarb Diet, which has been successful beyond my wildest expectations, was born. Now that I have been putting patients on this diet for about a decade, I am constantly amazed at how many people lose weight and keep it off, and it has absolutely nothing to do with exercise. It has everything to do with Addictocarbs.

One last comment on this matter. My favorite TV show, as you can probably imagine, is *The Biggest Loser*. I watch raptly every week as people lose weight and I remind myself of how far I have come. The most compelling part of the show is the relationship between the trainers and the contestants. The trainers exercise these people to exhaustion, cajoling them and exhorting them on. This show and shows like it have spawned a host of celebrity trainers, who have websites, health books, and lifestyle brands. Recently one of those trainers made some comments to the press:

> *Celebrity trainer Bob Harper, of the weight-loss TV show* The Biggest Loser, *has built a career putting very obese people through some grueling fitness paces but if he's learned anything from the experience, it's that diet trumps exercise every time . . . Gone are the days when he believed it was possible to just exercise the pounds away.*
>
> *"It is all about your diet," Harper, 48, said during a break from filming Season 15 of the long-running U.S. show. "I used to think a long time ago that you can beat everything you eat out of you and it's just absolutely not the case."*[1]

So the first weight loss myth is that you can exercise your way to being slim—you can't. The next myth I want to dispel is important because it is a basic element of the Addictocarb Diet.

FRUITS

The South Beach Diet is terrific and has gone a long way to explain the difference between many good carbs and bad carbs to the American public. However, I almost fell out of my chair when I got to page four of the book and read the lines, "For the next fourteen days . . . no fruit ever." How, I wondered, could that be part of this terrific diet, when in fact, on my diet, which I *know* has worked so well for me and my patients, eating fruit is at its very core?

South Beach is certainly not alone in forbidding fruit, even if only for the first fourteen days. In fact, an article in the *Journal of the American Medical Association* called "Effects of

Dietary Composition on Energy Expenditure during Weight-Loss Maintenance" states very clearly that very low-carb diets are the best for losing weight.[2] Of course, it does not say they are necessarily the best diets for your body or whether they are sustainable, but just that they work best for short-term weight loss.

So, low-carb diets work. But all of these diets exclude fruit simply because of all the carbs in fruit. How can that be, if I have lost sixty pounds, and my patients have lost untold pounds, by eating tons of carbs and calorie-laden fruits? Quite simply, a large part of the answer to that question is some misunderstandings about *fruits*.

Sophie Egan, in an article in the *New York Times*, makes the case for fruits.[3] She points out that fruits, in spite of having lots of sugar, are still good for you. She quotes doctors and studies supporting the fact that fruits do not get a fair shake.

Sure, fruits are good for you. Everyone knows that. They have anticancer properties. They have fiber that slows down the absorption of sugar and makes you feel full. They have antioxidant properties to help destroy those evil free radicals, and are rich in vitamins, minerals, and more good things. The US Department of Agriculture says, "Dietary fiber from fruits, as part of an overall healthy diet, helps reduce blood cholesterol levels and may lower risk of heart disease. Fiber is important for proper bowel function. It helps reduce constipation and diverticulosis. Fiber-containing foods such as fruits help provide a feeling of fullness with fewer calories."[4]

Okay, we get it; fruits are good for you. But the single most important reason that I think fruits are good for you has absolutely nothing to do with the advice of fruit cheerleaders, mothers, or even the US Department of Agriculture. The single most important reason for dieters to eat fruit is that it mitigates food cravings. It intercedes in the addictive potential of other foods. It is like cleansing your addictive palate—a mini-rehab. It resets your brain to ameliorate cravings. How do I know this? I have learned this through experience with almost a thousand patients. I am constantly gratified when I talk to a patient on my diet who tells me, "You know, it is funny, I just do not have the cravings anymore."

> The single most important reason for dieters to eat fruit is that it mitigates food cravings. It intercedes in the addictive potential of other foods. It is like cleansing your addictive palate—a mini-rehab. It resets your brain to ameliorate cravings.

One last thought on fruits that bears a mention: Fruit juice is not fruit. It is juice. It is the end result of squeezing all the sugar out of the fruit to make liquid sugar. Not only that, high fructose corn syrup is often added and the fiber is often entirely removed. Juice does not mitigate cravings, it causes them. No matter what it says on the bottle, it is not good for you. It is more like soda than fruit. So in case there is any question, when I say fruit, I do not mean fruit juice.

So there it is: You should exercise for your health, not to lose weight; and you should eat fruit for nutrition *and* to lose weight.

PART TWO:

The Diet

CHAPTER 4

Two Rules to Help You Lose Weight and Keep It Off

RULE #1: NO BREAD, NO POTATOES, NO EXCEPTIONS

We have already touched on the fact that what drives weight gain is craving certain foods I refer to as Addictocarbs. In Step 1, which encompasses the first three days of the diet, you will only be drinking Shakes, so obviously you will not be having any Addictocarbs. In Step 2, over the next two weeks, you will be allowed to eat some foods but, again, no Addictocarbs.

Why do you have to stay off all Addictocarbs for three days plus two weeks? Because you cannot be a recovering alcoholic, enter rehab, and have a beer every day. By the same token, you cannot start this diet, which is essentially Addictocarb rehab, and eat those evil Addictocarbs. Over time you will be able to add some Addictocarbs, but there are two Addictocarbs that are special—just two that deserve the distinction, in my experience, of being referred to as the worst Addictocarbs. In fact, they are so bad they have their very own rule. It is Rule #1 of the diet. So which ones are they?

They are the ones with the most addictive potential, and, frankly, you do not need to be any nutritional genius to figure which ones they are. Just look around and see what foods people are stuffing themselves with the most: bread and potatoes.

In fact, I was discussing this with the chief surgical resident at the hospital one day. She was just setting on a path to becoming a gastric bypass surgeon, and she inquired about my diet. Before I could say a word, she blurted out, "Just don't tell me I cannot eat bread and French fries." Of course, that was *exactly* what I told her.

Bread and potatoes are everywhere, in a million different forms, and are hawked mercilessly. Some forms of potato include French fries, baked potatoes, potato rolls, potato salad, home fries, mashed potatoes, potato chips, potato soup, potato skins, potato pancakes, potato gnocchi, and potato flakes.

Bread is even more ubiquitous: It is on sandwiches, comes as hamburger and hot dog buns, and sits there on the table in just about every restaurant in a bread basket. There is olive bread, raisin bread, sourdough, rye, pumpernickel, and cornbread. It often comes with butter or olive oil or fruit spreads. Pizza is bread with some sauce and cheese. Crackers are really bread that are just funny shapes and a little crispy. Bagels are bread. Bread pudding obviously has bread. Soup and salads come with bread. Eggs come with toast. Tortillas are really nothing more than Mexican bread, and they're present in tacos, quesadillas, and burritos. French toast is bread. And how many things are breaded and fried? There's even bread in store-bought meatballs and meat loaf. You get the point.

Even in minute amounts, bread and potatoes cause cravings. Just one French fry or one piece of toast will set them off. That is why this rule is so severe. I will introduce you to some bread and potato alternatives, though. Also, as you progress with your weight loss there will be room to negotiate a number of things, depending on how much weight you want to lose and how thin you want to stay. But one thing is totally nonnegotiable during the first two weeks of the diet and only seminegotiable after that: Rule #1, no bread and no potatoes.

It continues to amaze me at how easy it is to fall off the wagon. One piece of bread at a restaurant or a few home fries with breakfast and the cravings come rushing back. I have fallen off the wagon a few times in recent years. The worst was my most recent lapse, which caused me tremendous suffering and highlighted what I, as do all alcoholics and drug addicts, already knew was true—that it does not take much to fall off the wagon.

I was at a world-famous and very well-regarded restaurant in NYC. My wife and I were there as guests of a prominent gastroenterologist and his wife. Needless to say, we were very excited. We arrived at the restaurant at 6:15 P.M., and did not leave until 12:30 A.M. Over the course of the night, we were treated to some interesting conversation with the owner and chef, who expounded on the merits of his delicious *and* health-conscious cooking. It all sounded great, and as the meal progressed the food came out in waves of extremely small portions. I was thrilled that essentially everything that we were eating fit neatly into my diet.

As I sat at the table eating with my thin wife and the gastroenterologist's thin, former-model wife, I could not help but notice that everyone at the table except me was partaking of the stupendous-looking bread. Everyone seemed to be enjoying it and the waiter kept coming by and asking if anyone wanted more bread. I initially told him not to bring me any bread, so he just asked the others, who also said no. They were satisfied with their initial piece, and I was managing to not have *any* bread, because on my diet, Rule #1 is no bread, no potatoes. Then, caught up in the moment of the evening, as the waiter kept coming by and offering more new and interesting types of bread with each course, I relented. I had one small roll. Then I had another, and then another.

After that I noticed one dish had a minimal amount of potatoes in it and I thought, oh well, just this once and it's so little anyway. So I had it. Then I had more bread. My wife even asked if I should be having that much bread. I explained that it was a special occasion in one of the world's great restaurants, blah, blah, blah—the kind of blah, blah, blah-ing that a drug addict or an alcoholic uses to explain falling off the wagon.

Anyway, the night was great, we all had an amazing time, and it was perhaps the best meal of my life. It was also the best meal of my wife's life, though in her case she managed to get through it with an absolute minimum of bread.

I cannot deny that as we went home I was happy. I felt wonderful. I love food and this evening had been not only a great social experience but also a food lover's dream, an extraordinary meal at one of the world's truly great restaurants. I commented to my wife that while there must have been eleven courses, they were all tiny and quite healthy, and as a result I did not really feel stuffed. She felt the same way. But *she* didn't have six or seven pieces of bread. No, that would be me.

I awoke the next morning ravenous. Usually when I wake up that way, it is a clue to start the day off with a Shake. But this particular morning, I seemed to lack the usual control. I decided to have an egg omelet; not a bad way to start the day and it fits neatly into my diet. Ah, but this day was different. This was the day after the night I ate seven pieces of bread. This day, I thought I could just have a few home fries with my eggs. In fact, I felt *compelled* to have a few—the way an alcoholic is compelled to have a drink or a heroin addict is compelled to get a fix. I felt compelled, and I knew it was wrong, but I just could not help myself. "Big deal," I said. I had lost sixty pounds. Is a few home fries going to reverse that? Just like an alcoholic who says, "What is just one drink going to do?"

My wife noticed and said something. I pointed out to her not to forget that I had lost sixty pounds and kept it off for a good number of years. Certainly I could have a few home fries, no problem. She shrugged.

So I had a few home fries. Then I reasoned that since this was sort of a special occasion and the home fries were really, *really* good that day, I might as well finish them because I would not be having anything like this anytime soon. But "anytime soon" turned out to be lunch, which was only about two hours after breakfast. My lunch included a sandwich on two slices of extra-thin whole wheat bread, which even in my addiction-induced haze, I knew was wrong. And while I did not have fries with my sandwich, I did sample those of my lunch companion. No big deal. In retrospect, this is what the alcoholic says to himself after the *second* drink.

Without drawing this out any further, I went on a binge. It started slowly—just a few fries and whole wheat bread on a sandwich. I was soon eating bread and potatoes a few times a day. Then there was the occasional piece of cake. Then there was rice with Chinese takeout and oversampling the pasta I made for my son—not the Dreamfields pasta (see the section on Addictocarb Alternatives, page 147), which might have been okay, but fresh-made pasta I purchased at the local gourmet grocery store.

I could be a very sneaky eater, having had a lifetime's experience of food overindulgence. Also, it didn't look much different from the amounts I had recently been eating. When I ate home fries with eggs, it seemed like a regular portion. If I had some fries with lunch, it was just a small portion. But by the middle of the week it had moved to a medium portion, and by the end of the week, it was a large. Nevertheless, I went about my life, and everything seemed fine. I went to work and saw patients, and the occasional patient who had not seen me in a long time would come in and marvel at how thin I was. Yes, I explained, I had lost fifty pounds.

By the end of the week, after sitting down to a famously massive pastrami sandwich from the legendary Carnegie Deli in New York's Theater District, and after polishing off an equally massive piece of cheesecake, and then asking for another piece to go, I realized what was happening. In just a few days my cravings had all come back, and I was almost powerless to control them.

I was reminded of the scene in the movie *Chocolat* when the mayor of the town, who has tried to ban the bakery, loses his mind, breaks into the bakery, and in a fit of gluttony gorges himself on chocolate—only to collapse and fall asleep in the bakery store window, where he is found the next morning. Yes, that was me. I had gorged myself for a week and was experiencing the equivalent of waking up in the storefront window. I was a big hypocrite, on my way to becoming a big, *fat* hypocrite. I had broken my first rule by eating bread and potatoes. It is amazing that it took me a week to figure it out. I was on a bender—no different from an alcoholic. Of course, unlike an alcoholic, my addictive relapse was just not that apparent.

I came home that day with my cheesecake slice to go and the first thing I wanted to do was put it in the garbage. But I know myself; I am not above pulling it out of the garbage. So I opened the box, mashed the cheesecake up with a fork, ran it under the tap, made it into a gooey mess, and *then* threw it out. Then I did the single most important thing: I made myself a Shake. I sat down and drank and drank until I could drink no more. As I sat there, I heaved a sigh of relief. It was over, I thought. Then I weighed myself and found that I had gained nine pounds in a week. As is the nature of a food addict, I was starving. So I made a hamburger—no bun—and another Shake.

The next three days were not pleasant. I was literally overwhelmed with cravings, but I stuck to my plan, drinking three or four Shakes a day and eating salads and bunless hamburgers. I even had some Dreamfields pasta.

As I got into the third day, the cravings were beginning to subside. By the fourth day, I was sort of okay. Over the next few weeks I would have cravings again, but every time I did

I had a Shake. Finally, after about three weeks, it was over. I was back to normal. And it all started because of one piece of bread at a restaurant.

Looking back on it, I truly believe that I could have eaten that entire meal at that amazing restaurant minus the bread and been fine. I have tested out that theory by going out with the same couple to a few other exquisite restaurants. Each time the meal was great, but I kept to my basic Rule #1—no bread, no potatoes, no exceptions. I did not fall off the wagon again.

At one of those exquisite meals our friend, the gastroenterologist, said, "I've been gaining too much weight. How do you stay so thin?"

It's easy, I told him. Just stick with Rule #1.

RULE #2: DO NOT EAT *JUST* BECAUSE IT IS MEALTIME; ONLY EAT WHEN YOU ARE HUNGRY

I realize the idea of skipping any meal, and especially breakfast, is considered heresy in the general weight loss community. They insist that you should never skip breakfast because if you do, cravings will come later in the day and you will end up eating even more than you would have normally. While I will concede that eating later at night is worse than eating earlier in the day, I totally reject the notion that skipping breakfast will cause you to eat more later in the day. I have been telling patients for years that the only reason that people eat too much later in the day is because of cravings. If you eat Addictocarbs in the morning for breakfast, you will be hungry later in the day. If you do not, you will not be any hungrier later. So if you are not hungry in the morning, skip breakfast.

Recently this whole breakfast issue has come to the forefront in both medical literature and the media. An article in the *American Journal of Clinical Nutrition* studied the effectiveness of breakfast recommendations on weight loss and clearly concluded that "contrary to widely espoused views, this had no discernable effect on weight loss."[1] The *New York Times* picked up the story with an article titled "Is Breakfast Overrated?"[2] that stated, "For now, the slightly unsatisfying takeaway from the new science would seem to be that if you like breakfast, fine; but if not, don't sweat it."

Do not eat breakfast just because it is time for breakfast. Do not eat *any* meal just because it is mealtime. It is important to understand our cultural habituation to the "three meals a day" concept as opposed to daylong "grazing" when hungry and abstaining when sated. Eat only when you are hungry—including if you're in the middle of a meal. Ask yourself halfway through a meal if you are eating because you are hungry; if the answer is no, stop eating. If you decide you are still hungry, then continue eating, but constantly reassess your hunger. Keep doing this until you feel sated. It is just like filling up a gas tank in car.

A good tip that's been widely confirmed is that it takes about twenty minutes for your stomach to let your brain know that you are full. The more slowly you eat, the more likely it is that your brain will get the message to stop eating in time for it to do some good. "Leisurely" is the best pace for eating any meal.

If you are dining out, eat until you are no longer hungry and take the rest home. You'll not only lose weight and keep it off, but you'll also save money. The comedian George Burns was once asked how he stayed so thin despite eating most of his meals out. His answer is worth remembering: "Eat half." He lived past 100.

So as we get ready to take the plunge into the diet, let's just keep two overriding thoughts in our heads.

Rule #1: Under no circumstances are you to eat bread or potatoes at any time on this diet. If you have to fall off the wagon, just don't do it with bread and potatoes. That said, I will present you with bread and potato alternatives and even explain what to do just in case you *do* eat some bread and potatoes.

Rule #2: Do not eat any meal, even breakfast, just because. Only eat when you are hungry.

Now let's get started.

CHAPTER 5

Step 1: "Shaking" the Addiction

During the first three days you will not be consuming any Addictocarbs, but you will be consuming lots of carbs by consuming a detox drink I've created, which is known as the Shake. Remember that you will stick exclusively to these Shakes *only* for the first three days, because I have found that is the length of time required to break the cycle of addiction. For a complete list of what you cannot eat during Step 1, see Appendix B (page 205).

> During the first three days of the diet, you will eat only nutritious, tasty health Shakes. Nothing else. After that, other foods will be added, but for the first three days, nothing but my Shakes.

I want to be clear about one thing: The Shake is not the diet and the diet is not the Shake. It is only one part of a regimen to help you lose weight and keep it off. During the first three days of the diet—the "shaking the addiction" phase—the Shakes are a kick-starter. Think of this period as a transition between the old you and the future, permanently thin you. Later, the Shake will be something else entirely. You will use it to help maintain your slim figure, to quell cravings, or to rededicate yourself to the diet if you have fallen off the wagon. But for the first three days, it is the only thing you will be eating.

So why do I refer to the Shake as a "detox drink"? It is because I liken giving up Addictocarbs to giving up drugs or alcohol in a substance abuse program. I started calling it that as sort of a joke because everyone was asking me how I lost so much weight. "The Detox Shake," I would say in jest. Patients would ask what it was and how to make it, and I would tell them. They would then mention it to other patients. When they began to tell me they had recommended it to many other people who found it helpful, I became a little uncomfortable, because when *I* told a patient about the Shake, I would explain its place in my theories of cravings, Addictocarbs, and food addiction. It troubled me that people were recommending the Shake to other people out of context. I felt it was just wrong for people to think that only the Shake was my recommended way to lose weight. I needed to explain the entire program to people. This book is my way of doing so.

"THE SHAKE"
Yield: About 6 cups

Ingredients	Calories	Carbs (in g)
1–2 pints of strawberries or raspberries, or about 1 pound of mixed berries or other fresh or frozen fruits	160–320	38–76
¼, ½, or even 1 whole banana	32–130	27–136
3 ½ cups skim milk (or almond milk or soy milk)	360	50
1–2 pitted prunes	20–40	5–10
Optional: 2–4 scoops flavoring powder	220–440	60–120
Totals	**792–1290**	**180–392**

- Some great flavoring powder options include Slimfast®, Ovaltine, Whole Foods brand powder, and GNC brand powder; see my see my comparison of the various powders later in the chapter. Some people may not want or need a flavoring powder; if you leave it out, you will lose even more weight and lose it faster.

- Since you will be drinking nothing but these Shakes for three days, you might consider if it is easier to start the Shake regimen over a weekend, even though patients report that bringing it premade to work in a thermos is fine, as discussed below.
- You can still drink coffee, tea, and alcohol, because while I have issues with these, dealing with more than one addiction at the same time is just too much. If you have coffee or tea, you should not use table sugar, honey, agave nectar, or other kind of sugar-based sweetener. This is addressed further in the FAQ (Appendix A, page 191).

Throw all the ingredients in the blender. Blend on high for ten to twenty seconds. It should make about six cups. If you have a smaller blender, just cut the recipe in half. If you drink it all and you are still hungry, just make another one. Drink as much as you want. I keep one in the fridge at all times, just in case I get a craving. Blend it up, put it in a big portable container, and bring it to work with you. The less flavoring powder that you use, the less caloric it will be, but do not obsess over this. The important thing is to use as much as you need to feel sated. I use two cups of raspberries, half a banana, and three scoops of Slimfast®. Some patients have told me that they are fine without the banana or with zero, one, or two scoops of Slimfast. Sometimes they add three cups of strawberries. No matter how you make this Shake, you will lose weight.

While this is the basic recipe for the Shake, you can vary the types of fruits you use, or the quantity of the fruits, with each Shake for variety. I find that blueberries, blackberries, strawberries, and raspberries are best, but if you prefer other fruits like peaches, plums, or apples, that is fine, too.

Still, just looking at this recipe makes *me* nervous. Its calories and carbs are staggeringly high. How can it possibly work when the plethora of low-carb diets recommend daily carb levels of 20, 60, or 100 g per day? Is it possible to lose weight eating something like this? The answer is absolutely, positively yes. I have done this with almost a thousand patients and it works. I will explain how this can be true later in the chapter, in the individual sections on the Shake components.

One thing I will say is that there are many reasons why each component contributes to weight loss, especially the fruit.

So, how did the Shake evolve? I wanted to make a non-caloric health shake, thinking it would help me lose some weight. I started with half a banana, a few strawberries, and a scoop of Slimfast blended with two cups of skim milk. It tasted pretty good, but frankly I was still hungry, and it was not really sweet enough for me. So I added more powder and more strawberries. Soon I was using two pints of fruit and four scoops of powder, and mixing it in with almost a quart of skim milk. With this new recipe I felt sated and, strangely enough, noticed my cravings for Addictocarbs decreasing. I also noticed that my blood sugar was really good. I was amazed. Next, I noticed that I could drink as many Shakes as I wanted and my blood sugar was *still* fine.

Then the really big idea hit me. I was drinking a few quarts of these Shakes a day, my blood sugar had stabilized, I was not having any cravings, *and* I was losing weight. I sometimes left out the flavoring powder or the banana, and soon I was losing weight even faster because of the fewer calories—and the Shakes were still tasty. That is how this incredible weight loss journey began. Suddenly I was getting skinnier, and my patients were beginning to notice. They asked how I did it, and I was only too happy to share my success with them. I was as shocked as anyone when the patients began telling me how well the Shakes worked for them.

Suddenly I had a population to test the Shake on—my patients. And they were great. They would try the Shakes and report back to me. I was making charts and diagrams and began to research possible reasons that the Shake could be working. In doing my research, and putting it together with what I had learned about the Shakes from both myself and my patients, I developed my theories on Addictocarbs. It was then that I finally realized that you only needed to stick to the Shakes completely for a few days to shake the addiction. After that, with the help of the various Addictocarb Alternatives, you could just use the Shakes occasionally or in certain situations such as when going out to eat, falling off the wagon, or rededicating yourself to the diet, which I will discuss later.

Let's go through the components of the Shake and fill you in on some of the things I learned, including why they might very well lead to weight loss in spite of the high carb and calorie load.

FLAVORING POWDER

I want to make one thing clear: What makes the Shake so useful is the fruits, those craving-killing powerhouses of fiber, vitamins, and antioxidants. It has nothing to do with the flavoring powders. While I often use a powder for my Shakes, as do many of my patients, quite a number of them have gone out of their way to tell me that they prefer the Shake without it. For some patients, just the banana and other fruits provide them with all the taste they need. I think that is great. Like many of my patients, however, I prefer the Shake with flavoring powder.

The fact that some of these powders have sugar in them comes up, and I have already said you must cut out sugar. While some do have sugar, the ones that I use tend to have very little, as evidenced by their low glycemic index. Further, let's remember that not all sugar is bad for you. For instance, fruit has sugar in it but is still good for you, and you will still lose weight when eating lots of it on this diet. The fruit in the Shakes helps ameliorate even the very small amount of sugar you get from these powders. Let's examine some of them more closely.

I do not own stock in the companies that make Carnation or Slimfast. They do not pay me any money to promote their products. I use them because they serve my purpose. But you must bear in mind a very important point regarding branded powders. I *only* use these powders in the Shake.

I *never* recommend drinking the cans of premixed Slimfast or mixing these flavoring powders in milk or anything else. They have no place in this diet without the fruit. Also, keep in mind that not only can you simply leave flavoring powder totally out of the Shake, but you can also substitute a number of different ones and the diet will work just as well. Examples that I have studied include Optifast, Medifast, Carnation Instant Breakfast and No Sugar Added Breakfast Essentials, Chocolite, generic protein powders from GNC, Whole Foods' 365 protein powder, Proventive, Garden of Life RAW Protein, Ovaltine, and a variety of powders sold on Amazon.

I reviewed the various flavored powders, checking them for efficacy on the diet and taste, comparing and contrasting the various components, and came up with some interesting facts. Some are meant for weight loss, some for muscle building. Some are health food store protein powders; others are an instant breakfast drink with or without added sugar. One is a popular children's chocolate drink flavoring that touts its lower sugar content. I used chocolate flavoring because that is my favorite flavor, but the other flavors are all basically the same in makeup.

My findings were as follows:

Taste: The winner for taste hands down was Slimfast, so this was the one I used to measure all the other types against. Carnation Breakfast Essentials No Sugar Added was a very close second, and Optifast was pretty good, too. The various health store protein powders generally were less palatable, some much less, but they tend to be less caloric, with a lot fewer carbs and, of course, lots of protein. My nurse uses one of these generic powders, and she likes it and has lost a lot of weight.

Carbs: When evaluating their carb content, try to stick to ones that have fewer than 20 g of carbs per serving— the lower the better, assuming you like the taste. Even if it has very few carbs, you won't drink it if you don't like it! Just to mention, Carnation Breakfast Essentials No Sugar Added has 12, Ovaltine 10, and Slimfast 18 carbs. The various protein powders had the lowest carb counts, but at the expense of taste.

Sugars: The protein powders had the least sugar in them, but again at the expense of taste. In general, try to stick to powders that have less than 10 g of sugar per serving. Carnation Instant Breakfast No Sugar Added has only 7 g. Slimfast has 10 g, which is half of Carnation Instant Breakfast Regular, but a lot more than the protein powders and Medifast. The Whole Foods brand has less than 3 g per serving. Check your labels and balance it with taste.

Fiber: An extremely important parameter is fiber content because it can serve to lower the glycemic index of the other ingredients, and Slimfast has a very good 4 g of fiber. Chocolite and some of the other protein powders are quite good on fiber, as is Carnation Breakfast Essentials No Sugar. Ovaltine has zero.

BERRIES

I primarily use berries in my Shake, even though you can use other fruits like peaches, apples, and mangoes. I like berries because they are nutritional powerhouses that taste great and prevent cravings. An essential component of the berries and other fruits I use in my Shake are antioxidants. So I just want to say a few words about them and free radicals before I proceed to discuss the fruits of the Shake.

Antioxidants and Free Radicals: A Classic Story of Good and Evil

Like most stories of good and evil, the pairing of antioxidants and free radicals is not all black and white. Free radicals are occasionally helpful to the body, sometimes traveling around helping the body defeat viruses and infections. But then the body has to get rid of the free radicals. If the body is unable to do so, they can cause havoc by damaging other cells.

You can get free radicals from lots of things, like cancer, smoking, or exposure to toxins in pesticides or pollution. X-rays cause free radicals; so do stress and alcohol consumption. These free radicals can attack cells, which may cause them to function poorly or even die. This cellular damage is a common pathway for a host of pathological conditions. Many authorities believe that aging is caused by a buildup of these free radicals. Along with the medical professionals who believe that you can get free radicals from cancer, many believe that they cause, or at least exacerbate, cancer. LDL—the bad cholesterol—is also impacted negatively by free radicals.

Under normal conditions the body can handle a certain amount of free radicals. But sometimes the body becomes overwhelmed and needs help to fight them off. That help comes from antioxidants.

Antioxidants are always the good guys in this story. It is their job is to go around the body neutralizing free radicals so that they do no harm. The interesting thing from the point of view of this diet is where you get antioxidants. The simple answer is fruits and vegetables.

Tufts University famously ranked[1] the various foods that have a lot of antioxidants. Blueberries, prunes, strawberries, cranberries, blackberries, raspberries, and apples all made the top twenty, with six of the top twenty fruits ending in "-berries." It's no coincidence that these are the most important components of my Shakes.

Strawberries

I love strawberries. They are one of my favorite foods. They taste good, they are easy to grow, they cleanse your bloodstream of lipids after eating meat, and they decrease food cravings. In short, they are really, really good for you.

It is impossible to miss the constant stream of articles proclaiming the health benefits of strawberries. Articles like one from the *British Journal of Nutrition* proclaiming that strawberries reduce blood glucose[2] are just music to my ears. Of course I want to lower my blood sugar. All diabetics do. That they may also help prevent against esophageal cancer[3] piques my interest as well, since that runs in my family.

The most interesting claim from the point of view of this diet is that strawberries may stimulate metabolism and suppress appetite.[4] I already know that they suppress cravings, but it is nice to know that there is some science to corroborate my beliefs about a whole slew of their potential benefits.[5]

Strawberries may help improve heart health, lower the risk of developing some cancers, and reduce blood pressure.[6] They may also be somewhat anti-inflammatory, since studies have shown that they lower C-reactive protein, which is a blood marker not only for heart disease but also inflammation. Thus they also may help with arthritis.[7]

BERRIES AND BURGERS

Strawberries are always good, and so are burgers. Strawberries and burgers together are an interesting story. Some research shows than when you eat a burger, combining it with strawberries may actually help to cleanse the body of lipids from the burger. Of course it sounds more impressive when you say, "Strawberry modulates LDL oxidation and postprandial lipemia in response to high-fat meal,"[8] which was the finding of a 2010 study, but to put it simply, strawberries are good for you, especially when combined with meat. So any time you have a burger or other beef, why don't you just have a few berries with that burger? I do.

Of course, strawberries also contain a good amount of carbs and calories in the quantities I use. In a Shake, I usually use between one and two pounds unsliced, or about 3 ½ cups, which adds up to about 200–250 calories and 55 g of carbs. It sounds like a lot, but it does not raise my blood sugar, which goes along with what these articles have said.

One of the great things about strawberries is their availability. You can get them year round from somewhere, and very often organic are available. One of my friends who is a gardener also assures me that strawberries, raspberries, and blackberries are really easy to grow, so you can have them fresh from your garden as well.

Last, this is one food you can easily get frozen and even frozen organic. My favorite frozen organic fruits are from Cascadian Farms,[9] and two packages total twenty ounces, which is exactly the right size for one of my Shakes.

Raspberries

I think I made my point on strawberries by quoting articles, books, and medical studies, so I am not going to bore you with all the same stuff about raspberries, but let's just say they are really good for you, too. Raspberries have lots of vitamins, fiber, and antioxidants that go a long way toward keeping the body healthy by gobbling up free radicals. They may protect against macular degeneration and cancer. They are a low-glycemic food and have riboflavin, niacin, folate, potassium, magnesium, calcium, vitamin A, copper, iron, lutein, and plenty of vitamin C. The frozen kind is easily found and is just as good as the fresh, and, once again, I always try to get organic, because I am nervous about pesticides. My favorite frozen organic raspberries are Cascadian Farms.[10] Just as with strawberries, two packages of Cascadian Farms raspberries equal twenty ounces, exactly the right size for a Shake.

PRUNES

One fruit I should mention in a special context is prunes. I understand that they are just dried plums, but the important thing for me is that they tend to thicken the Shake, which I find quite pleasing, and they add non-Addictocarb sugary sweetness for taste. Remember, this is the good kind of sugar—not all carbs are created equal. Prunes have a very low glycemic index and will not raise your blood sugar or cause cravings.

The aforementioned Tufts study ranked prunes very high on the list of fruits containing helpful antioxidants. And I could not end the discussion of prunes without at least mentioning their legendary salutary effects on colon health. But you get the point; prunes, just like almost all fruits, are very good for you.

BANANAS

Everybody loves bananas. Everybody knows that these delectable fruits have lots of sugar, carbs, and calories. How can you lose weight on these? Let's consider a few things here.

According to the USDA National Nutrient Database, a banana between seven and eight inches long contains 26.95 g of carbohydrates but less than .39 g of fat and only 1.29 g of protein. Bananas are very high in potassium: A medium banana has 422 mg, along with 32 mg of magnesium and 26 mg of phosphorus. It also supplies about 10.3 mg of vitamin C and contains valuable amounts of A and B vitamins as well. The nutritional value of bananas in various stages of ripeness is the same and so is the energy. A medium banana has about 90 calories. Two medium bananas equal approximately one cup.

The Banana Diet was created by Sumiko Watanabe, a Japanese pharmacist from Osaka, for her husband. He lost thirty-seven pounds on the diet. It became so popular in

Japan around 2008 that it even led to a temporary shortage of bananas there. The diet recommends eating bananas for breakfast and more throughout the day. It is still popular in Japan, and there are always articles in other places about people trying it successfully. So if bananas are a high-calorie, high-carb food, how can this be possible? It *is* possible; you can eat bananas and lose weight. How, you wonder?

Bananas are a good source of dietary fiber, both soluble and insoluble. Two bananas have 6 g of fiber. Fiber makes you feel full because of its bulk in the gastrointestinal tract. Also, fiber is absorbed very slowly and drags some excess calories along the intestines with it, before they can get completely absorbed. Supposedly, there is resistant starch in the bananas that ferments in the digestive tract and creates by-products that increase fat burning by 20 to 25 percent. Some believe that the resistant starch consumption may even decrease fat accumulation.[11] I am sure about one thing: You can eat bananas and not get fat, so you can put half a banana or more in the Shake. End of conversation.

MILK (COW, ALMOND, OR SOY)

I only use organic skim cow's milk. Some people use 1 percent and the occasional dieter uses 2 percent, though the lower the percent the better. I caution my patients to stay away from whole (4 percent) milk. However, it does not always have to be cow's milk. Some patients use almond or soy milk for a variety of reasons, such as allergies, lactose intolerance, or simply wanting to adhere to a plant-based diet. Lactose-free soy and nut milks are extremely important in the African American community, as well as with the elderly.

One cup of skim milk has about 90 calories and 12 g of carbs and has a relatively low glycemic index. It is a good source of vitamins and nutrients, containing protein, vitamin B$_{12}$, selenium, vitamin D, riboflavin, calcium, and phosphorus.

A large percentage of its calories come from sugars but that is okay; I will discuss this further a little later.

All sorts of benefits have been claimed for milk, from being good for your skin (supposedly Cleopatra took milk baths) to being good for your muscles. My son, a competitive runner, drank milk before and after each race. I think many of us can remember being given a warm glass of milk by our mothers to help us fall asleep. It may be beneficial to your eyesight. Everyone knows that it promotes healthy bones, especially if it is fortified with vitamin D, but the most important thing for our purposes is that it has been advanced as promoting weight loss, especially in women.

A number of articles have suggested that milk is weight loss Nirvana. One article from the *British Journal of Nutrition* clearly states in its title that "milk supplementation facilitates appetite control in obese women during weight loss."[12] Another article states in its title, "Increased consumption of dairy foods and protein during diet- and exercise-induced weight loss promotes fat mass loss and lean mass gain in overweight and obese premenopausal women."[13] The articles go on and on. Of course, for every article promoting the weight loss properties of milk, there seems to be one refuting it.[14] How do you decide based on the conflicting research? I can only say that I have recommended milk to people, especially women, to aid weight loss for a long time, and it seems to work. It is essential in the Shake and is a good source of protein, which I believe leads to satiety.

But a very large question looms here. What if you cannot drink cow's milk because of allergy or lactose intolerance? Also, what if you are opposed to drinking milk because, for instance, you prefer a plant-based diet? There are numerous substitutes that are also referred to as "milk," and many of my patients have used them effectively. Almond milk and soy milk are only two examples. Other nut milks are beginning to hit the market. You can even make your own.

Soy and almond milk differ from cow's milk in some ways, such as taste (almond milk is sweeter). Their calorie and carb contents differ somewhat (soy milk is about the same as skim, and almond less). Cow's milk has more protein. Despite the differences, the important thing to me is that, whatever milk you use for the Shakes, they will help you beat your addiction to Addictocarbs.

So, after three days of Addictocarb Detox, drinking nothing but Shakes, it is time to move on to the next phase of the diet: Step 2, Addictocarb Rehab.

CHAPTER 6

Step 2: Beginning Addictocarb Rehab

This step will last two weeks. During this time you will stay off all Addictocarbs, which again are *bread, potatoes, pasta, flour, rice, sugar, high fructose corn syrup, fruit juice, and soda.* Remember: I have chosen these nine *specifically* because over the years, in treating my many patients, I have found that *these* foods and ingredients present the greatest addiction challenges. Let me be clear about this list. While you should not have *any* of these Addictocarbs for these two weeks, I will give you alternatives for bread, potatoes, and pasta. Let's touch on these foods briefly before we go on to the foods that you *can* eat. There is a complete handy list in Appendix B on page 205, but here is a very brief discussion of the main components.

Bread and potatoes: Remember Rule #1: no bread and potatoes. If you need reinforcement, just reread chapter four. Bear in mind that pizza is bread with stuff on top of it. Wraps and pitas and tortillas are out. Avoid meatloaf or meatballs unless you know they were made without bread. Avoid breaded anything. When in doubt, check ingredient labels.

Flour: Nothing that is made with flour. This includes things like baked goods, which are generally loaded with flour and sugar—cakes, muffins, donuts, cookies, scones, pies and other pastries, and pretzels. There is often flour in breakfast cereals. Wheat flour is also used to make a roux as a base for thickening gravy and sauces. You cannot have it. Also avoid anything battered with flour, like fried chicken and chicken fried *anything*.

Rice: No rice of any kind, though in the next phase you may decide to add to your diet an Addictocarb Alternative, such as kasha or quinoa or wild rice (which is not really rice), or even an Addictocarb Accommodation like brown rice.

Sugars: When talking about sugars, we need to understand that sugar sometimes gets a bad rap. Strawberries have sugar, and so do apples and other fruits, but they are not simple sugars, and the fiber in fruit serves to counter some of its bad effects. White table (granulated) sugar and brown sugar are both simple sugars, and they count as simple sugars whether they're in a cake recipe, scooped into your coffee, added to whipped cream, or in the maple syrup you put on your pancakes. When you buy food, check the ingredient list for added sugars and generally try to buy the product that has the least sugars in it.

One question that comes up is the matter of sweets, such as chocolate, ice cream, and breakfast cereals. There is not much to be said here. You cannot have them in the first two weeks because they contain sugar. Dark chocolate has more antioxidants and less sugar and has been shown to be beneficial in many ways, but it is still chocolate. Chocolate is also addictive in its own right, and you do not want to trade one addiction for another. Later you will be able to have dark chocolate, but not for these two weeks.

Ice cream has sugar, and you cannot have it for these two weeks.

Breakfast cereals deserve a special mention because they are so omnipresent. They are generally loaded with sugar and often made with white flour—and remember that all flours are off limits for this period. Stay away from breakfast cereals.

High fructose corn syrup: This is a tough one because it is everywhere—juice, cocktails, soda, breakfast cereal, yogurt, salad dressings, breads, baked goods, candy, condiments, soups, and nutrition bars. Be vigilant about avoiding it by checking the ingredients.

Fruit juice: Remember that fruit juice is not the same as fruit. We touched on this in chapter three. No fruit juice. It is bad for you. It is nothing more than liquid sugar. Fruits are good carbs, whereas fruit juice is an Addictocarb. A food item that uses fruit juice as a sweetener does not make it good for you.

Vegetable juices are fine, but watch out for the sodium content.

Soda: Soda, like fruit juice, is just liquid sugar. No soda. It is evil. Same for diet soda because it just fools your body into thinking it is sugar.

SO WHAT *CAN* YOU EAT?

First of all, check the detailed chart in Appendix B, the dos and don'ts of foods. There are certain foods that you *can* eat during these two weeks, no problem. For those that are not permitted, I will go over some reasonable, patient-tested alternatives that *are* permitted.

There are plenty of foods you can eat. You can drink the healthy Shakes and eat all meats, fish, and poultry. For a more vegan palate, you can have tofu, tempeh, and seitan.

You are welcome to enjoy all fruits, vegetables, legumes, nuts, cheeses, salads, and Addictocarb Alternatives for pasta, bread, and potato. One thing you will not miss on this diet is variety.

WHAT *CAN* YOU EAT?

- SHAKES
- PROTEIN (meats, fish, and poultry)
- FRUITS
- VEGETABLES
- LEGUMES
- NUTS
- CHEESE
- SALADS
- PASTA ALTERNATIVES
- BREAD ALTERNATIVES
- POTATO ALTERNATIVES

(see the dos and don'ts list in the appendix)

To stave off Addictocarb cravings, you need to do two things: Eat some high-calorie, non-Addictocarb carbs, and eat some protein. Let's discuss these briefly.

Protein

Protein is important because it helps to satiate hunger. How you get the protein is up to you. Chicken, meats, fish, nuts, beans, cheese, eggs, and tofu are the most common choices.

Since the proteins are being used to quell hunger, you should only eat as much as you need. As this diet progresses, you will find you will need less and less. One very good way of eating only as much as you need is what I call the "quarterburger" strategy.

The Quarterburger Strategy: I make hamburgers (no buns) and cut them in quarters—hence the term "quarterburger." If I am hungry I will have a quarterburger with my Shake or meal. If I want another quarterburger, I have it. In the beginning you may need to have four quarterburgers or even more. As you progress, you will find that you may be able to do with fewer and fewer quarterburgers.

Quarterburgers are handy. You can wrap them in plastic wrap and throw a couple in your purse or your briefcase (refrigerate if you need to keep them for more than three hours). You can eat them throughout the day. If you prefer chicken as your protein source, then just imagine a quarterburger's worth of chicken, but the concept is the same. You can eat a quarterburger piece of steak or tofu or cheese. The important thing here is to only eat as much as you need.

Shakes

You can have a Shake any time you want. In fact, the more Shakes the better. You should make at least one Shake (about 6 cups) per day and keep it around in the fridge, in a thermos, or at work, to head off cravings and hunger. One Shake a day is a good starting point. I cannot emphasize too strongly how important the Shakes are. They are nutritious and quell the cravings.

Fruits

You can eat whatever fruits you want because they are not Addictocarbs. However, I would keep certain things in mind. Pineapples, watermelon, and dates are relatively high in calories and have easily absorbable sugars; while they do not cause cravings, their sugars are not good for diabetes. Bananas are acceptable in the Shakes, because after all, you can only consume so many bananas in Shakes, but eating a banana every half hour around the clock is going to add up to lots of calories. The same is true for avocados; in moderation (no more than one avocado a day) they are fine.

Vegetables

You can have vegetables—any vegetables—but they cannot be breaded. Eggplant parmesan is fine as long as the eggplant is not breaded. Vegetable tempura is off limits because it is coated with flour, which is an Addictocarb.

Salads

Make your salads with oil and vinegar dressings. Other dressings may be okay, but you must check the labels to make sure they are not full of sugars or high fructose corn syrup. If a regular salad does not satiate you, then why not try my son's special burger salad in the recipe section (page 135)?

ADDICTOCARB ALTERNATIVES

What are Addictocarb Alternatives? These are foods that I have compiled over the years that fit neatly into the framework of the Addictocarb Diet. They often resemble the Addictocarb that they replace, like "mashed cauliflower" instead of mashed potatoes. They do not induce cravings, and can sometimes suppress them. I have recommended these foods to my many patients over the years, and their feedback has been invaluable in evaluating them. Some of the foods are simple and self-explanatory; others have an interesting story, like Dreamfields Pasta.

THE PASTA ALTERNATIVE

Dreamfields Pasta

Pasta is my favorite food, and quite frankly, I am not sure how I would survive without Dreamfields pasta.

While pasta is an Addictocarb, *this* pasta is not. Why? Because this company has done something ingenious, so that it will *not* cause pasta-like cravings, it will *not* cause an Addictocarb-like increase in blood sugar, and it will *not* cause weight gain. Most important, it does these things without changing the taste and the texture of the pasta. Let me explain.

Dreamfields has come up with a way to make pasta that renders the carbs much less digestible. It is beautifully explained on the company's website,[1] but the gist is that while it is made of the same ingredient as regular pasta (durum wheat semolina), it contains an added mix of harmless fibers and wheat protein[2] that set up barriers to digestive enzymes. These ingredients make the pasta more difficult to digest, making it functionally more like fiber. If you do not digest the pasta, then you don't gain weight, it does not raise your blood sugar, and it will not cause cravings. With Dreamfields you will get only a fraction of the cravings associated with regular or whole wheat pasta. Is it perfect? No, but it is close.

There are still some caveats with this, which are also true of traditional pasta: The longer you cook it, the more caloric it becomes and the more likely it is to raise your blood sugar. The pasta should be cooked *al dente* (Italian for "to the tooth," meaning pasta should have some "bite" to it).

When I first heard about this pasta, I was incredulous. I had tried every whole wheat pasta on the market and every low-carb pasta that I could get my hands on, both boxed and fresh. With each pasta that I tried, I would meticulously and obsessively check my blood sugar every hour; all of them raised my blood sugar unacceptably. Then I found Dream-fields. I was dumbfounded when I saw my results; it simply did not spike my blood sugar.

The last thing I want to say about this pasta is that it is— to my taste—indistinguishable from regular pasta. I was the only one in the house watching my blood sugar and the only diabetic, so I would make this pasta for myself and continue to make the regular pasta for my wife and kids. Then they all tasted Dreamfields and found it comparable to regular pasta, to the point where I no longer make them separate pasta. I began to recommend it to my patients, and I was astounded at their comments. They were telling me that they loved the taste; furthermore, they were not experiencing cravings.

Other Pasta Alternatives

There are some people who, for a variety of reasons, cannot eat Dreamfields pasta, and they have mentioned to me that they have had better luck with pasta made from Jerusalem artichokes, which strangely enough are neither from Jerusalem nor related to artichokes. In fact, the Jerusalem artichoke is made from something called sunroot, a species of sunflower, originally cultivated in North America by Native Americans. It is sometimes used as a substitute for potatoes or animal feed and, of course, in pasta. While somewhat high in calories, it is still an extremely healthy food because of its high fiber content, minerals, electrolytes, and antioxidants. It does not seem to cause cravings like regular pasta and has been shown to be very good for diabetics. I have tried it; it seems quite tasty and only has a slight effect on my blood sugar. While I accept that it may work, I just do not have the breadth of experience with this as I do with Dreamfields, so if any of the readers find that it works, or that other alternative pastas like quinoa pasta and the various nut flour and bean flour pastas work, please drop me a line on *The Addictocarb Diet* website at http://www.Addictocarb.com.

THE BREAD ALTERNATIVE

Wasa® Crisp'n Light 7 Grain Crackerbreads

These are crackers that take the place of bread, and they do it quite well. They are made with whole-grain wheat, wheat, rye, yellow corn, barley, spelt, whole-grain amaranth, and quinoa. This product is all natural, does not contain trans fats, is a good source of whole grains, and, almost unbelievably, contains only 20 calories per slice. (If you need a gluten-free version, try Natural Nectars Cracklebred®.)

I have tested this carefully on myself and found that it does not raise my blood sugar significantly. I also found that it does not induce cravings. I have recommended this to countless patients who have reported that it works for them, too. Many have become fanatical about it. You can get it in most supermarkets, but I just order it from Amazon by the case.

I use this exactly the same way that I would use bread. I use it to make cheese sandwiches, peanut butter sandwiches, turkey or ham sandwiches, or any other kind of sandwiches (my favorites are raspberry and peanut butter sandwiches). Patients have told me they use it like bread crumbs in dishes like meatballs or meatloaf. I put it on the table just as I would have normally put out bread, and I eat it with soups. I break it up and use it as croutons for salads. I even dip it in olive oil, just like great Italian bread.

Lettuce Wraps

While technically this is not a bread alternative, it can be used in certain cases in place of bread. You simply use large leaves of romaine lettuce in the place of bread, tortillas, or buns. As we will see later in the fast food section, some burger places like Carl's Jr. and Hardee's use it to sandwich their burgers when you request a bun-free burger. The lettuce provides a crisp, refreshing texture, works well with a variety of fillings, and is gluten free.

Cucumber Chips

While I realize that cucumber might sound like an odd bread alternative, I do believe that it can function quite well to replace things like tortilla chips or other chips for dipping in things like salsa, guacamole, and hummus.

THE POTATO ALTERNATIVE, OR THE SWEET ALTERNATIVE TO KILLER POTATOES

I am passionate about sweet potatoes. That may sound odd. Used as a potato alternative, sweet potatoes will help eliminate cravings and help you lose weight. For me there is another truth. Sweet potatoes have been instrumental in helping me conquer my diabetes.

Sweet potatoes are a relatively high-carb, high-calorie food that fits nicely into the Addictocarb Diet. They are low in sodium and very low in saturated fat and cholesterol. Sweet potatoes are a good source of dietary fiber, providing double the amount of fiber of white potatoes. They also have about half the glycemic index of white potatoes, which is extremely important for diabetics. They have potassium, vitamins A, B_6, and C, and manganese. They are also a great source of antioxidants, which, you will remember, are really good for you. Most important, sweet potatoes do not cause the kind of addictive behavior regular potatoes do. They do not stimulate the addiction center of the brain, and as a result do not cause the same cravings.

They can be prepared in most of the same ways as regular potatoes: fried, baked, mashed, even baked as chips and grated for pancakes.

If you are thinking that one of the most difficult forms of potato to give up is French fries, I am with you on that one. I love French fries. Fortunately, over the past decade or so there has been an explosion of the availability of sweet potato foods, especially fries. While a few years ago virtually all hamburgers came with regular French fries, I now find that you can get sweet potato fries almost anywhere. That includes fancy restaurants, takeout places, and food fairs. You can even buy them frozen in the supermarket. I am not sure exactly why this has happened, but this is a real boon for the Addictocarb Diet.

Aside from how well they facilitate weight loss with the Addictocarb Diet, sweet potatoes are great for diabetics. I am not reinventing the wheel here. I know that many articles explain how good sweet potatoes are for diabetics, but for me it is intensely personal. As I have mentioned, I am compulsive about checking my blood sugar, sometimes checking it up to ten times per day. After eating regular potatoes, my blood sugar usually spikes to about 300, which is a danger zone. I have checked my blood sugar after eating all kinds of sweet potato recipes, and repeatedly my reading actually goes down, usually to the very low 100s, which is very close to normal. Some have suggested that this is because adiponectin, a hormone produced by fat cells that is typically low in diabetics, is raised by eating sweet potatoes. Whatever the reason, I know from personal experience that sweet potatoes work for treating diabetes as well as for weight loss.

After years of being on the Addictocarb Diet, I am still surprised and exhilarated when I take my blood sugar after eating sweet potatoes.

Now let's move on to Step 3.

CHAPTER 7

Step 3: Staying Slim for Life

This step should ideally last for the rest of your life. The single most important thing about this step is not just the addition of new Addictocarb Alternatives and Accommodations (which I'll get into later), but rather the sense that you will be making decisions about how to live the rest of your life. You will need to come to some internal understandings of what is right for you.

In my own case, I knew that I needed to lose more than fifty pounds, so I stayed on the diet for quite a long time. Over the past ten years I have found a steady point. My weight fluctuates situationally. For example, I may be going on vacation, out to dinner, or to a wedding. When I do this, I keep my decision making uppermost in my mind. I do not fret when going out to dinner where I know I will be tempted to consume Addictocarbs. I have the security of knowing that if I do, when I get home, a Shake will be there for me when the cravings hit. I think of the Shake as an old friend.

Some things will change in Step 3 and some things will stay exactly the same as Step 2. For a complete list of what foods are okay during Step 3, see Appendix B (page 205).

Drinking the Shakes stays the same. You will still drink them as often as you can. The Addictocarb Alternatives introduced in Step 2 for potatoes, bread, and pasta are the same.

What is new in Step 3 are additional Addictocarb Alternatives for rice. Also new are Addictocarb Accommodations, which help you deal with the Addictocarbs you are just not willing, or not ready *yet*, to give up.

As mentioned, the most important thing about Step 3 is that it is decision time. Now that you have lost some weight and quelled your cravings, you will have to decide how much more weight you want to lose and how badly you want to keep it off. Do you need to lose another thirty pounds? Do you only need to lose ten pounds? Have you lost enough weight, and do you just want to maintain your new contours?

Let's face it, whether you want to lose more weight or just keep off what you have already lost, you are going to have to give up something. The decision of how many somethings—and how much of each something you give up—will be up to you.

Going forward, for every single Addictocarb that you give up, you will lose that much more weight. If you give up bread only, you will lose weight; sacrifice just potatoes and you will lose weight; give them both up and you will lose even more. Throw rice and flour into the mix of things you give up and you'll be better still; let go of high fructose corn syrup, fruit juices, and sodas and even more weight will stay off.

While I do not mean to belabor the point, the reason the Addictocarb Diet works is because it decreases cravings for Addictocarbs. You do not have to give up all Addictocarbs if you do not want to, but the ones you choose to give up must be given up totally and completely. No, you cannot have just a thinly sliced piece of bread, or a half a piece of bread, or whole wheat bread, or any other kind of bread. You cannot have a few French fries, or just a small piece of cake, or just one small glass of fruit juice. In most diets this whole "eating in moderation" thing purportedly works in the short run; however, it *doesn't* in the long run. Just a quarter slice of whole wheat bread stimulates the addiction center of the brain. To avoid that stimulation you must stay off bread completely. If you fall off the wagon, then you acknowledge it and deal with it, but you simply cannot delude yourself into thinking that by just limiting an Addictocarb you will be able to stay slim. You won't.

Those who treat alcoholics know about the "slippery slope" principle. Some alcoholics go through detox and rehab and then return to real life. Pretty soon they convince themselves that they have their addiction under control, and wouldn't it be nice to have just one glass of white wine or one bottle of beer a day? One glass becomes two glasses, then an entire bottle or six-pack, and finally a full-blown binge. It's the same with Addictocarbs. Telling yourself you can have French fries once a week is a slippery slope back to obesity. Once you start stimulating those addiction centers in the brain, your cravings will overwhelm you.

In Step 3 you will get to make your decisions with another Addictocarb Alternative added to the mix. This time the subject is rice. You couldn't have this alternative in Step 2, but in Step 3 you may, in addition to Addictocarb Alternatives for pasta, potatoes, and bread. Granted, rice might be the one Addictocarb you choose to live with, but before you make that decision, I urge you to try the rice Addictocarb Alternatives.

Let's talk about these new choices, and then we will discuss the decisions you have to make.

RICE ADDICTOCARB ALTERNATIVES

Kasha and quinoa are Addictocarb Alternatives to rice. Let's discuss these one at a time.

Kasha

Kasha is a high-calorie, high-carb Addictocarb Alternative to rice that is nutritious, protein packed, gluten free, and delicious. It would be banned by many low-carb diets. Three-quarters of a cup of prepared kasha has 170 calories and 35 g of carbs. It is high in fiber and antioxidants and is an excellent source of protein.

Kasha, or buckwheat groats, is technically not a grain, even though it looks like, tastes like, and has the texture of a grain. It is technically a fruit or a seed. In a culinary sense, however, it is a grain and, like rice, can even be boiled or steamed. You can use it as an accompaniment to foods just as you would use rice, and you can use it as a bed on which to put things like pot roast, shish kebabs, and fish. You can eat it with stir-fried vegetables and in soups.

Quinoa

The United Nations General Assembly declared 2013 as the "International Year of Quinoa."[1] Quinoa has been a staple for thousands of years in the Andes region of South America. It is usually considered to be a whole grain, though it is actually a seed, and it can be prepared like a whole grain and substituted for rice. It has higher protein content than most whole grains and provides all essential amino acids, making it a complete protein. Quinoa is gluten free and cholesterol free. One cup of cooked quinoa has 220 calories, 3.5 g of fat, 5 g of fiber, 40 g of carbs, and 8 g of protein.[2]

From the standpoint of this diet, quinoa serves as an excellent Addictocarb Alternative for rice. Like many of the things on this diet, it has lots of carbs and calories, but it is a good Addictocarb Alternative because it does not cause as many cravings or as big a rise in blood sugar compared to rice.

Like rice, it is very easy to prepare; you simply cover it with water or vegetable stock and boil until soft for about fifteen minutes. You can even cook quinoa in a rice cooker, which, as far as I am concerned, is poetic justice. You can also use it as a breakfast cereal, similar to oatmeal. I have a number of recipes in the recipe section on ways to prepare quinoa (pages 155–158), but the bottom line is that it is an Addictocarb Alternative for rice and can be used in any way that you can use rice.

One further point is that quinoa also comes in pasta form and so can be used as an Addictocarb Alternative to pasta (though in truth it pales next to Dreamfields in terms of taste and texture).

Now that we have discussed the Addictocarb Alternatives to rice, it is time to bring up the concept of Addictocarb Accommodations.

ADDICTOCARB ACCOMMODATIONS

Perhaps you are thinking, "Meet me halfway, Doc. I really don't want to give up rice/pasta/flour." The Addictocarb Accommodation is me meeting you halfway in Step 3. You might not lose as much weight or as quickly, and you'll have a bit more of a struggle keeping it off, but before you consider going back to white rice, semolina pasta, and white flour, try to acclimate yourself to these Accommodations. For rice the Addictocarb Accommodation is brown rice; for pasta it is whole wheat pasta, and for flour the Addictocarb Accommodation is whole wheat flour.

The important thing to understand about these Addictocarb Accommodations is that they *do* cause cravings, and although they *are* fattening and they do raise blood sugars, they are not as bad as their white counterparts. So you must decide how much weight you want to lose and let that decision guide you in deciding whether to stay at Step 2 a bit longer, or to enter Step 3 and make choices in light of your new Addictocarb Alternative and Addictocarb Accommodation options.

DECISIONS

When it comes to people making decisions on their weight loss prerogatives, I have a perspective based on my experience with patients. I have found that when I explain the concept of Addictocarbs to patients they listen intently, but as soon as I mention *giving up* Addictocarbs their eyes glaze over, their bodies tense, and I lose their attention. The concept of giving up all Addictocarbs is just too overwhelming. However, when I point out that they can start with giving up *only one* Addictocarb and they will lose weight, they breathe a sigh of relief, relax, and start listening again. That is why as patients enter Step 3, I always ask them one important question. It is the same question I ask of you, the reader. Take a moment to reflect before you read on. Are you ready? Here it is:

Which one Addictocarb is your worst enemy? Pick one from among *bread, potatoes, pasta, flour, rice, sugar, high fructose corn syrup, fruit juice, and soda*. Write it down right here:

> **MY WORST ADDICTOCARB FOOD**
>
> _____
>
> _____
>
> _____

I then tell the patient to give up that one Addictocarb and nothing else. Of course, you can still have Addictocarb Alternatives and Accommodations, but you need to pick one Addictocarb to give up completely.

I can tell you from dealing with patients over these many years that getting a patient to give up just one Addictocarb works. When I tell this to my patients, their usual response is, "Only one thing, I think I can do that." I have been pleased by how many patients have lost weight by just giving up one Addictocarb, if it is the right one. Let's face it, if you decide to give up pasta and you actually rarely eat pasta, it will not help. You must give up the one that causes you the biggest problem. What I have found is that once people are able to give up one, they will eventually be ready to give up another, and then another. My Addictocarb Choice Tool will help make this easier for you.

The Addictocarb Choice Tool

Use this to determine which three Addictocarbs are your worst enemies and ultimately which one is the absolute worst. The amount of weight you will lose on the Addictocarb Diet will be determined by how many Addictocarbs you give up totally. After you have successfully given up one Addictocarb, you can move on to the next, and the next one after that. Some people can do very well if they only give up one Addictocarb, especially if that one is their worst offender. If you can give up three Addictocarbs, your weight battle will be mostly won. If you have diabetes like me, you may need to give up most, or even all, Addictocarbs.

The Addictocarb Choice Tool

Pick three foods from this column that you feel you crave the most and list them in the next column.	After you have listed three foods from column 1 below, pick just one food and list it in the next column. This should be the number one food you crave.	Here is the worst Addictocarb and the one you should probably give up if you are only going to give up one.
Bread		
Potatoes	1 _____	
Pasta		
Flour*		
Rice	2 _____	_____
Sugar		
High fructose corn syrup		
	3 _____	
Fruit juice		
Soda		

* If flour is too big a category, you can just pick things like cookies or cake.

Everyone is different, and everyone has different Addicto-carb addictions, but I have found that if you are going to start with only one Addictocarb, then the most effective one from a weight loss perspective should be either bread or potatoes. Still, for some people, it may be another. So the biggest decision you will need to make in Step 3 is which *one* Addictocarb is your worst addiction and commit to yourself that you will banish it from your diet.

If you feel you can banish two or three Addictocarbs, all the better. But the reality is that it is better to pick one Addictocarb and work at eliminating it from your diet than to try to banish four Addictocarbs and fail at all of them. It is important on this diet, as it is in most things in life, to meet with success. You should start with easily attainable goals. Giving up just one Addictocarb is a great place to start.

LOSING THE BURDEN OF ADDICTION

I am exhilarated by the feeling that I am no longer in the throes of addiction. It is a tremendous feeling of freedom and accomplishment. Even after being thin for the past ten years, I still get that feeling. It is the feeling of a free man who was once enslaved. I have spoken to other addicts about their past addictions. They, too, are relieved to be free of the burden of feeling compelled to indulge their addiction, though they are forever wary of the way back.

The simple act of walking down the cookie aisle of a super-market and not feeling compelled to buy some is to me a true definition of freedom. I can say to myself that I am still an addict, but I also know that I have overcome that tremen-dous pull that I have suffered with most of my life. I realize now, in retrospect, the agitation I used to feel while walking down those aisles—the need to buy something addictive, get home, and rip the bags open. That compulsion is gone. Sure,

I sometimes get a little wistful, and when I do I just have a Shake or a bowl of strawberries.

The potato chips aisle was always a tough one for me. As I pass by them, I smile to myself and feel a sense of satisfaction, the same sort of satisfaction as when I think of an old girlfriend. I wish them my best, and while I will occasionally have a wistful thought about them, I am quite happy that it is only a passing thought. I remember the old heartache, but it is not so bad anymore because I am in a new, much healthier relationship.

I can walk by an open-air restaurant and see people eating French fries. I see the mountains of bread stacked in baskets on their tables. It still looks and smells wonderful, but I do not get that underlying gnawing that I must have some. I remember how gratifying it used to be, and know that it could be so satisfying again, but I know that it could never really work out between us. I know that the relationship we had was just too self-destructive. So I just smile, take a deep, satisfied breath, and walk on by. I am enthralled by how I have moved on to new relationships that may be less intense, but far more satisfying.

I have found that Step 3 is where patients seem to come up with the most questions. As a result, in the FAQ section, I have compiled a list of questions from patients that are either most frequently asked, or that I thought were really insightful. I also welcome any further questions, which you may ask on my website at http://www.Addictocarb.com.

I have found that the most commonly asked questions about the diet are not about the diet itself, but rather falling off the diet, so I will address that issue first.

CHAPTER 8

Getting Back "On the Wagon"

WHY DO YOU FALL OFF THE WAGON?

Addicts will fall off the wagon. They are addicts and that is what addicts do. Some popular diets have their own ways of dealing with this. Certain diets have daily or weekly point systems that pace your indulgences over the course of a day or week. Other diets advise portion control. Some diets even suggest that you can make up for your excesses by fasting, either regularly or intermittently. All of these "solutions" just skirt the real issue of *addiction*. They fail to take into account that the addiction center of the brain has been stimulated; how you deal with *that* will determine your ultimate diet success.

I do not delude myself, nor do I allow my patients to delude themselves. I accept the reality of my addiction, and I am clear with my patients about that reality, too. I accept that my lifetime of being overweight had its roots in addictive behaviors. When I fall off the wagon, I am just like any other addict. What do I need to do? I need to get myself straight again. I always explain this to my patients while gently reminding them to view their diet relapse through the lens of addiction.

People fall off the wagon for all sorts of reasons, real and imagined: weddings, graduations, holidays, travel, work-related dinners—even just falling prey to the aroma of French fries or pizza. It happens all the time, and how you deal with it will ultimately determine your overall success on the diet. It is no big deal. Just go on the Shakes for a day or two and make sure not to break Rule #1: no bread or potatoes. Then get back on the diet. As long as you view your diet relapse in the context of an addiction, then you will have an easier time getting back on track.

An important question keeps coming up about what to do when you feel that you will be exposed to addictive substances, such as dining out, which is a challenge to anyone on a diet. What steps can you take to minimize the impact of dining out on your diet? While it may sound almost counterintuitive, it is actually what you do before and after the addictive event that is most important.

WHAT STEPS CAN YOU TAKE TO MINIMIZE THE IMPACT OF DINING OUT?

I get this question all the time from patients. I have a dinner engagement on the weekend but I really want to stick to the diet—what should I do? In fact, I have a handout in my office that I give to patients when they ask. Here it is:

THE ADDICTOCARB DIET
Dining Out Handout

1. Have a Shake or a bowl of strawberries (or other fruit) before you go out to eat.
2. Absolutely *no bread and no potatoes* at dinner.
3. IF you are hungry after the main course, have fruit for dessert, or at least a dessert that has fruit in it.

If you completely refrain from all Addictocarbs, it ends here; if not:

4. Have a Shake when you get home from dinner.

5. Have a Shake the first thing the next morning.

6. If you continue to have cravings, keep having Shakes until the cravings subside.

Prior to going out you should drink a Shake, even if it is only a small glass of it, or eat a bowl of strawberries (or other fruit). This will make you far less hungry and thus less likely to fall off the wagon. The last thing you want to do is to show up at a restaurant starving. That is just an open invitation to devour the bread basket. During dinner, the single most important rule is to stay away from bread and potatoes, though the fewer Addictocarbs you eat the better.

One way to deal with this is what my friend Larry refers to as "bread basket geography." He sends back the bread basket or parks it as far from himself as he can, and, if all else fails, he will at least move it to a location on the table where it is obstructed from view. While I appreciate his strategy and accept its usefulness, I believe it becomes less and less necessary the longer you are on the Addictocarb Diet. The whole point of the Addictocarb Diet is that if you stay off Addictocarbs you will not feel the pull of addiction. As one patient told me, "When they put the bread on the table, I am amazed that I have absolutely no desire to eat it." I feel the same way.

Here's another useful suggestion: When the waiter comes over to get your drink order, ask your server to bring an Addictocarb-free appetizer with the drinks. If the entrée comes with potatoes, ask the waiter to substitute sweet potatoes or virtually anything else for it. For dessert, try to stick to fresh fruit or at least with desserts that have fresh fruit in them.

You will find that the longer you are on the diet, the less of an addictive pull you will feel. As one patient said to me, "I was at a meeting yesterday. When they broke out a box of cookies, there was nothing about it that was appealing to me." I hear this a lot from patients, and it just echoes my own personal battle with food addiction. This emphasizes how people feel when they conquer their food addiction by staying on the Addictocarb Diet.

In case, for one reason or another, you weren't able to follow these suggestions and fell off the wagon, the next most important thing is what you do after you get home. You need to detoxify. You can have a Shake or a bowl of strawberries or some Addictocarb Alternative of your choosing, whether you are hungry or not—even though it goes against my tenet of only eating when you are hungry, because there are exceptions to every rule. In a sense it cleanses the addictive palate. No matter how much I ate when I was out, or how full I was when I got home, I almost always wanted to eat more. And I did. Funny thing, though, after drinking a Shake or eating a bowl of strawberries, I was not in the mood to finish off my leftovers or have a late-night snack.

The morning after is the single most dangerous part of falling off the wagon. If you have been out and had a few pieces of bread or some French fries, you must be aware of the fact that you have now stimulated the addiction center of your brain and you *must* intercede to prevent a cascade of addictive events known to alcoholics as "going on a bender." First and foremost, you must quell the cravings. You need to take in large quantities of calories and carbs that are *not* addictive. You can do this by eating fruit, or any of the Addictocarb Alternatives, or simply having a Shake. In my experience treating patients, I've learned that Shakes seem to be the easiest way of quelling the cravings, though personally I always reach for a bowl of strawberries. So the first thing you do in the morning, or whenever it is that you will next eat, is to have a Shake or some fruit or some Addictocarb Alternative.

It is okay to fall off the wagon temporarily, but you just need to detoxify and get back on track again.

How long should you stick to detox? For me, it is usually two days. For some people, it will be less, and for some people it will be more. Part of that has to do with how long you have been living the Addictocarb Diet lifestyle. If you have been on the diet for two weeks, two months, or two years, you will have different experiences getting back on the wagon. I can tell you from personal experience, as well as from speaking to almost a thousand of my patients, that the longer you are on the Addictocarb Diet, the easier it will be to stay on it and deal with the occasional lapse. I cannot remember the last time I had an Addictocarb, and I hear similar comments from many of patients. I just do not feel the pull of addiction any longer, and neither do they.

TIPS FOR STICKING TO THE DIET ON VACATION

One "falling off the wagon" question comes up very frequently: What about vacations?

When I go on vacation I always do one interesting thing: I always purchase a small hand blender—nothing fancy, they usually cost less than ten dollars—and make Shakes in the room of wherever I'm staying. This is especially easy if you are staying in hotel suites with kitchens or in hotels that provide mini-fridges instead of minibars. Call the hotel ahead of time and ask about this; you'll be surprised at how many will accommodate this request.

My friend Larry has yet another strategy. He and his wife tend to stay at economical all-inclusive resorts, which are quite popular. These usually offer buffet meals, and so Larry and his wife graze the buffets for Addictocarb-free foods. These establishments typically offer a wide selection of fruits, vegetables, salad fixings, and a variety of proteins, all of which fit into the Addictocarb Diet. I am told that sweet potatoes are also beginning to show up at these buffets more and more often.

PART THREE:

Daily Living and The Addictocarb Diet

CHAPTER 9

Gluten Free, Lactose Free, Vegetarian, and More

I get many questions about lifestyle and the Addictocarb Diet. For example: What if I am vegetarian, vegan, lactose intolerant, gluten free, need an anti-inflammation diet, or even a kosher or halal diet? Sometimes these diets are a matter of principle and sometimes they are born of medical necessity. Let's call them "lifestyle diets."

Throughout the book I touch on these issues when discussing lactose-free milks or making sauces and soups with and without animal protein. While it is difficult to go on any special diet, it is certainly no more difficult to stick to the Addictocarb Diet and observe special dietary considerations. Just to put it in some perspective, I will just discuss a few here.

GLUTEN SENSITIVITY

It has been clear to me for a good number of years that there are people who come up negative for gluten sensitivity or celiac disease on all hematologic and even endoscopic diagnostic tests, yet who could actually benefit from a gluten-free diet. As a result, I often suggest a two-week trial of a gluten-free diet to people suffering from a range of medical problems. I have seen it work particularly for people with gastrointestinal issues, but sometimes it has worked for fatigue, arthritis, behavioral and psychological issues, skin rashes, and migraines. Sometimes it works and sometimes it doesn't. In this day and age when it is so easy to get gluten-free everything, I figure that if you try it for two weeks and it helps, good; if not, there is nothing to be lost but a couple of weeks on a healthy diet.

While the Addictocarb Diet does not pretend to be totally gluten free, it is certainly what is referred to as gluten aware, which has come to represent a diet that restricts most but not all gluten. This is becoming increasingly important because many in the medical community now believe that you do not have to have celiac disease to suffer from gluten-caused symptoms. There is even a new classification called "non-celiac gluten sensitivity." In fact, Dr. Arthur Agatston noticed that many of his patients who initially did extremely well on his South Beach Diet started feeling poorly again when they got into the later phases of the diet. He reasoned that this was because he allowed slow introduction of gluten, so he actually wrote another book about it. Of course, they would not have had this problem if they were on the Addictocarb Diet because it is already gluten aware and just a hop, skip, and jump from being fully gluten free. The vast majority of gluten comes from wheat flour, which is prohibited on the Addictocarb Diet by virtue of excluding bread and flour.

Read labels carefully. Glutens, like sugar, sneak up on you through the ingredients of a variety of foods you might not suspect: many sauce mixes, bouillon cubes, gravies, breakfast cereal (even wheat-free ones), ready-to-cook flavored rice dishes, soy sauce, candy, chips, baked beans, and salad dressing. Even beer, Communion wafers, and some medications and vitamins. The one that really gets me is stamps and envelopes, so don't lick them if you are gluten sensitive.

LACTOSE INTOLERANCE

Lots of people have lactose intolerance. In the United States, some ethnic and racial populations are more likely to have lactose intolerance than others, including African Americans, Hispanics, Native Americans, and Asian Americans. The condition is least common among Americans of European descent,[1] supposedly because their ancestors lived where dairying flourished and passed on gene mutations that maintain production of the lactose-digestion enzyme, lactase, into adulthood.[2] But lactose intolerance is also very common in people with irritable bowel syndrome and Crohn's disease, which some suspect may actually just be lactose intolerance.[3] The lay literature is rife with claims that lactose causes all sorts of issues, most commonly diarrhea, flatulence, and abdominal pain, along with other conditions less often associated with lactose such as constipation, arthritis, sinusitis, and acne. Over the years, I have often mentioned giving up lactose to patients and in some cases it has helped tremendously.

My point here is not to discuss the state of the medical literature on lactose intolerance, or even to support or debunk the lay literature, but only to point out that if you feel that lactose intolerance is an issue for you, the Addictocarb Diet can still help you. As I mentioned in chapter five, you can always replace cow's milk with a nondairy option, which has worked for many of my patients.

WHAT IS A VEGETARIAN?

A vegetarian does not eat meat, fish, or poultry, and vegans do not eat their by-products, but the definition is not always black and white:

- **Semi-vegetarian:** A person who cuts back intake of meat, fish, and poultry.
  - A pollo-vegetarian avoids red meat and fish but eats chicken.
  - A pesco-pollo-vegetarian avoids red meat but eats chicken and fish.

- **Lacto-vegetarian:** Vegetarian who eats milk products.
- **Ovo-vegetarian:** Vegetarian who eats egg products.
- **Lacto-ovo vegetarian:** Vegetarian who eats milk products and eggs.
- **Vegan:** A vegan is the purest type of vegetarian, avoiding all animal products and by-products, even non-food items such as wool, silk, and leather. Some even avoid honey.

VEGETARIANISM

I mentioned in chapter one that if you want to go on a really great diet, you will do best eating mostly kale, Brussels sprouts, spinach, and broccoli. While I like all of these things to an extent, and recommend them to my patients, I would be insincere if I said that I try to observe this in my own life, or that I actually expect my patients to stick to this kind of diet. Yet it is no more difficult to be a vegetarian on the Addictocarb Diet than it is if you're not avoiding Addictocarbs. If you eat a plant-based diet, using nondairy milks in the Shake works perfectly well and perhaps even a little better for weight loss than cow's milk. In the recipe section there are things like the Cauliflower Pizza (page 137), which uses a cauliflower dough and could easily be made with soy cheese. You can also make the bean soup with a vegetable base instead of meat. And while I have two recipes for meat-based bolognese sauces, I also have one tomato sauce, my favorite, that is pure vegetarian.

Last, the Addictocarb Alternatives are by and large plant-based foods, as are the Addictocarb Accommodations.

ANTI-INFLAMMATION DIET

In terms of inflammatory illnesses, which are basically anything that ends in "-itis" and include such things as asthma, colitis, psoriasis, and even heart disease and dementia, I will only say that any list of anti-inflammatory foods will have berries at the very top of the list of good things to eat—and they are a mainstay of the Addictocarb Diet.

The Addictocarb Diet will easily fit into any lifestyle diet. If you have a specific question not answered in this book, please post your inquiry on my website: http://www.Addictocarb.com.

CHAPTER 10

Fast Food the Addictocarb Diet Way

I t's easier to follow a diet when you work from home, have no spouse or children, and rarely go out to socialize. But for most of us the real world is often at odds with our best dieting intentions. Hungry children, coworkers on a budget, spouses who are tired and just want that Big Mac right now—all conspire to undermine our efforts to lose weight and stay thin. So I set out, with the help of my nurses, present and former, and a few other people in various locales, to check out what happens at the intersection of the Addictocarb Diet and the fast food establishment. We tested places like Mexican restaurants, burger joints, sandwich shops, and smoothie chains.

While I believe that whole food, plant-based diets are generally healthier than most other diets, I also accept the reality that people are going to visit fast food establishments, and in order for a diet to be successful there must be considerations for fast food. This chapter is my attempt at that.

While places like Subway and Chipotle are very popular and can make it pretty easy to stick to the diet, burgers and fries are still the kings of fast food, and I do not believe that any diet can be successful unless you can weave these components into the fabric of a diet. As it turns out, it is actually quite easy to find burgers, and in some cases even fries, that fit neatly into the Addictocarb Diet, so let's start there.

BURGERS, SANDWICHES, AND MEXICAN FOOD

I like fast food as much as anyone, but I was astonished at people's reaction at the mere mention that I needed some volunteers to check out how the Addictocarb Diet would work at fast food establishments like McDonald's and Burger King. From their response, you would have thought that I was a casting director for a TV reality show on the Food Network. One of my nurses, Nicole, could not wait a *minute*, went out to McDonald's that day, and brought back some fascinating and useful information.

As I sent out more volunteers, it became clear that if I wanted to do it the right way I would need a number of people checking out restaurants in several locales. So I started with my nurses, present and former: Nicole in New York; Mandie, now a nurse practitioner in Missouri; and Donna, now a nurse in Indiana. As information began coming in, I mentioned the interesting results to a few patients. Soon I had people in Colorado, California, South Carolina, Florida, and even Spain and England chiming in with their results. The process was becoming unwieldy, and it was apparent that I needed to standardize the experience to get the best data, so I wrote up a very simple questionnaire for everyone to fill out in order to be fair to the various establishments.

It quickly emerged that some places adhere to the Addictocarb Diet better than others. What follows is the summary of the various evaluators' findings. I would be interested in what the readers of this book have to offer on this issue. Please post your thoughts on my website: http://www.Addictocarb.com.

Some General Points

The same thing was ordered at every fast food burger establishment: a burger without a bun. The counter staff was generally very helpful. While some places were more familiar with some of the Addictocarb concepts, the counterperson was virtually always more than willing to ask a manager to investigate if there was anything they could do to help.

None of the fast food evaluators except for Energy Kitchen seemed to have any luck finding sweet potato fries. This is in spite of the fact that numerous restaurants have either had them at one time, claim to have them at some locations, or supposedly test market them periodically. You will generally have much more luck finding sweet potato fries at regular restaurants.

Last, before reading this section, reread the "Berries and Burgers" box on page 55.

Carl's Jr./Hardee's

In general: Counterpeople were unperturbed, and since there is actually a low-carb option on the menu, most of the counterpeople seem to be up on it. What arrived was a box containing a hamburger without the bun, with mayo, mustard, tomatoes, ketchup, onions, pickles, and cheese *neatly sandwiched* in two lettuce leaves.

Addictocarb verdict: Excellent! Carl's Jr./Hardee's really get it when it comes to avoiding Addictocarbs. You get the regular burger experience without the bun. They go out of their way to make the burger still seem like a sandwich by substituting lettuce leaves for the bun. This is brilliant and convenient. While they do not have sweet potato fries, they have experimented with them in the past, and one can only hope that one day soon they will come back to it. Some of the testers' comments were:

- "Very satisfying since [there was] so much lettuce—it was more filling and pleasing to the eye."
- "It appeared like you were getting a meal instead of just a burger."
- "The sandwiching with the lettuce was great."

Burger King

In general: Burger King is supportive of Addictocarb principles. Technically, they have a "gluten-sensitive menu," or what they refer to as a "low-carb option." That being said, not all of the counter folks are that informed of it, but with a quick check with the manager it can easily be worked out. In one place, the counterperson was perplexed, but a simple shout-out to the manager got an "Oh, low carb, no problem" in return. In another location, they simply said, "Oh, we have a gluten-free option, no problem." The burger arrives in a small plastic container with pickles and ketchup on top, generally well presented and sometimes in a lettuce sandwich.

Addictocarb verdict: It is a true Burger King experience, just without the bread, but you should probably order the burger specifically by name, like "Whopper with cheese"— just without the bun. You might have to mention to the counterperson to check about the "low-carb option"; if that fails, just ask the manager. Also, Burger King has had sweet potato fries, but not at every location and not always—and even if they do, the fries might have sugar on them, so be mindful of that.

McDonald's

In general: A plain burger was ordered; it was delivered in a chicken nuggets box, and the counter staff was always matter-of-factly courteous.

Addictocarb verdict: McDonald's will accommodate no-bun orders very nicely if you order correctly. If you go into McDonald's and order a plain burger, that is exactly what you will get, bun and all. It is probably best to just order, for example, a Big Mac without the bun. So will McDonald's work with the Addictocarb Diet? Yes. In any case, it tastes like a McDonald's burger.

Sonic

In general: A burger without the bun was ordered, and the employee was very attentive, asking about ketchup, mustard, mayo, and utensils. It comes neatly wrapped in tin foil, lettuce and tomatoes carefully placed underneath.

Addictocarb verdict: Sonic is a pretty good place to get a burger on the Addictocarb Diet and generally provides a pleasant and efficient ordering experience.

Wendy's

In general: A burger with no bun was ordered, and that is exactly what came in a small plastic container with pickles, tomato, lettuce, ketchup, mayo, and onion. Counter staff always seemed overly helpful.

Addictocarb verdict: If you like Wendy's, you will like this burger. This is a great place to go if you want to stick to the Addictocarb Diet.

Energy Kitchen

In general: Sirloin burger with no bun was ordered, and they acted like they had been there before. I did not feel like I was the first person that had come in requesting no bun and baked sweet potato fries. The sirloin burger, cooked medium well, was delivered in a nicely covered bowl with pickles, tomato, onion, and special sauce. Unlike most of the other places, they not only have sweet potato fries, but they actually bake them instead of deep-frying them.

Addictocarb verdict: Virtually perfect. Burger was excellent, sweet potato fries were baked and fantastic, and the ketchup was organic and high quality. Best all-around fast food restaurant for the Addictocarb Diet.

Subway

In general: The Subway experience was remarkably similar from state to state and location to location. Perhaps that is because they make a big thing with Jared Fogle, the "Subway Guy," and how much weight he lost. They will make any sandwich as a salad without so much as the blink of an eye. It is clearly something they get asked a lot. Because of the great feedback that I received from around the country, I decided to check it out. I had a meatball parmesan hero as a salad. I thought it was great, and I was able to stay away from any bread, so I was able to have an Addictocarb-free meal.

Addictocarb verdict: Virtually perfect.

Chipotle

In general: Chipotle prides itself on being the healthy alternative to fast food. To a certain extent this is true, but it requires some simple choices on your part. Chipotle offers a variety of ingredients and will put whatever you want into your burrito or taco. By this time you know that the wrapping of a taco or burrito is an Addictocarb, so you can't have it. On the other hand, the "bowls" are very popular. This is where they put the ingredients into a bowl so that it is more like a salad—exactly the same, just without the Addictocarbs. Be careful, though:

If you want to stay away from Addictocarbs, leave out the rice, which is not really that big a trade-off in my estimation.

Addictocarb verdict: Virtually perfect. Overall, it is extremely easy to eat here and stick to your Addictocarb Diet guns.

FAST FOOD SHAKES

The importance of Shakes to the Addictocarb Diet is obvious. I understand there are a variety of circumstances where making a Shake is inconvenient or impossible. What do I do and what do I tell my patients to do? I get a Shake in one of the many shake and smoothie places popping up all over the United States. I have a place that I prefer, and patients have told me about places they prefer. Patients have also gotten these shakes at their health clubs. I will just mention a few here so you get an idea how easy it is to find these places.

Pinkberry

In general: This is one of my favorite places. It is one of many frozen yogurt stores now gaining popularity in the United States. They have more than 170 stores internationally, including more than 100 in the United States. Pinkberry serves frozen yogurt, which is relatively low in sugar, and they smother it in all types of toppings. This works well with the Addictocarb Diet as long as you stick to fruit and nut toppings instead of candy, but Pinkberry is of interest because they can truly make you a Shake. I have them use bananas, strawberries, raspberries, and blueberries; they then add fat-free milk and some yogurt, either Greek style or regular. Greek yogurt is less fattening, but either way this meets all the basic requirements of the Shake. If I am at my office, I can just walk over to a Pinkberry and have them make it. It works fine on the diet and I cannot tell you how many patients have told me that this works for them in a pinch.

Addictocarb verdict: Virtually perfect.

Health Club Shakes

In general: Just about every health club makes what they call health shakes. They generally consist of a protein powder, fruit, and fat-free milk. This is a perfect Addictocarb Diet Shake; just make sure they do not add fruit juice.

Addictocarb verdict: Often good but you need to pay attention to what they put in.

Juice Generation

In general: This place astounds me. Every time I go to one of these places, I cannot believe the number of people standing in line waiting for shakes. To get an Addictocarb Diet Shake, ask for fruit, fat-free milk, and a flavored protein powder and they will be happy to accommodate.

Addictocarb verdict: Virtually perfect.

Jamba Juice

In general: This chain has more than 800 locations. It is essentially a smoothie outlet, though they also sell food. Peruse the menu, speak to a counterperson, and you can easily get a shake that approximates the Addictocarb Diet Shake.

Addictocarb verdict: Often good but you need to pay attention to what they put in.

So, what have we found at the intersection of the Addictocarb Diet and fast food? The bottom line is that if you want to lose weight and stay thin, you are going to have to go out of your way somewhat to do it. But there are fast food alternatives that make it easier for you to stick to the diet. My survey, while not exhaustive, certainly made this very clear. Places like Chipotle and Subway make it very easy for you, but even burger joints like Burger King, McDonald's, Sonic, Wendy's, and Carl's Jr./Hardee's try to be accommodating. There are a plethora of smoothie places that will accommodate you, too. Check out the Addictocarb website (http://www.Addictocarb.com) to post your ideas and for further news on other fast food establishments and how they work with the Addictocarb lifestyle.

CHAPTER 11

Addictocarb-Friendly Snacks

What exactly is a snack? Is popcorn a snack? How about a sandwich or cherry tomatoes? How about a steak?

The dictionary defines a snack as "a small portion of food or drink or a light meal, especially one eaten between regular meals."[1]

Just about anything can be a snack. In my opinion, there are two kinds of snacks: the ones you eat because you are hungry and the ones you eat for fun.

If you are starving and need a snack to tide you over, there is nothing better than a protein. My favorite way to eat protein snacks, and one which my patients have embraced, is the quarterburger concept discussed earlier in chapter six.

If you cook a hamburger and sit down to eat it, you will eat the whole thing; but if you just eat a quarter and reassess whether you are still hungry, you will be surprised at how often you can stop at only a quarter or a half. Even if you eat three quarters of a burger and you decide that is enough, you still save 25 percent of the total calories. It adds up.

These things work perfectly in my diet as snacks. Why? The point of my diet is that you should never be hungry. Since I am hungry a lot just by nature, that means I have to keep eating all the time, and I do. I eat all kinds of proteins, but I just do it in chunks of quarterburger-concept foods.

While the second type of snacking is done to sate hunger to some degree, it fits more into the fun category. Let's face it, everyone wants some snacks while sitting in front of the TV and watching the ball game. How about when watching a romantic comedy, or a real nail-biter of a movie, or just when sitting around a campfire? Snacks in these situations are more for fun.

I have often wondered what makes a snack fun. The question that comes up is what, according to my diet, works to satisfy this desire? Here is my take on snacks. Popcorn seems to me to be the perfect snack. It is fun to pop in your mouth and chew, is high in fiber, has a relatively low glycemic index, and does not cause many cravings. Plus you can only eat so much popcorn. The same can be said for peanuts and a variety of other things.

So what snacks can you have on my diet? You can have anything that is not an Addictocarb. Popcorn and nuts of any kind are not Addictocarbs, and so you *can* have them. Just remember that popcorn or nuts with sugar on them *are* Addictocarbs, so keep that in mind if you are considering Cracker Jacks® or honeyed nuts.

One of my favorite snacks is cherry tomatoes. I have recommended them to people over the years as a good snack to have around, and have often been met with incredulous stares, only to be told months later that they have worked out wonderfully. Cheese cubes are also great. Berries of any kind—strawberries, raspberries, and blueberries—are not Addictocarbs, so they also make great snacks.

If you need to set out snacks for a party or a game, why not cut Wasa Crisp'n Light 7 Grain Crackerbreads cut into quarters and put them out? Forget chips, pretzels, cookies, candy, crackers, et cetera. You can't have them. If you do you, forget staying thin.

There are many Addictocarb Alternatives that you will find satisfying as a snack. Patients tell me about new ones every day. Yet one snack stands above all others and deserves some special attention here.

CHOCOLATE

I cannot tell you how many times, over the years, I have told a patient to go on a diet, only to have them tell me that they can never give up chocolate. If you feel this way, the good news is that on Step 3 of the Addictocarb Diet you can have chocolate in moderation. A discussion on chocolate is in order because it is among the most popular of all snacks, and it has many health benefits.

It appears from anecdotal reports, as well as some legitimate medical studies, that dark chocolate decreases cravings and promotes satiety. A Danish study published in the *Journal of Nutrition and Diabetes* in 2011 makes the point that health food enthusiasts have been making for years: "Dark chocolate promotes satiety and lowers the desire to eat something sweet."[2] This is totally in line with the basic premise of the Addictocarb Diet, that a strategy aimed at diminishing cravings is the only way to lose weight and keep it off. This study merely confirms what anecdotal reports have been saying for years. Dark chocolate decreases cravings. They go on to point out that this is especially true compared to milk chocolate.

However, you need a basic understanding of the "percentages" of cacao, the basic ingredient of chocolate. In short, the higher the percentage, the darker the chocolate, and the darker the better. For example, if you go into the Godiva Store you will see they sell one-inch square chocolates, some with 50 percent cacao, others with 72 percent. Keep to those with 72 percent. At the very least, the cacao needs to be above 60 percent. Milk chocolate, which is not good for you, is often down in the 50 or 30 percent cacao area. In fact, when you add milk to the mix, it negates almost all of the good effects of the chocolate.

So to the question, "Can you have dark chocolate on the Addictocarb Diet?" the answer is yes. What kind and how much? We can be safe in saying a one-inch square, or one ounce or so per day, is a reasonable amount. But there is a caveat. If you are going to eat chocolate, you should make sure that you are not adding extra calories. If you eat a lot of chocolate, you will gain a lot of weight. So try to cut something out of your diet of equivalent calories.

If you do eat chocolate while on the Addictocarb Diet, there are many health benefits that you may enjoy. First, chocolate is good for your blood pressure; cocoa phenols in the chocolate tend to lower blood pressure.[3] Chocolate also has flavonols, which are powerful antioxidants. Chocolate is one of the most powerful antioxidants, beating more well-known antioxidant powerhouses, such as green tea, wine, fruits, and vegetables.[4] We have discussed the good effects of antioxidants previously, and that antioxidants are the allies that protect you against those evil free radicals. The more antioxidants you get, the better; you can get them from fruits and vegetables, but you can also get them from dark chocolate.

Here are some of the other benefits of moderate use of dark chocolate:

- It stimulates the release of endorphins, those elusive and magical substances that make us all feel better about everything. "Runners' high" is supposedly the result of the release of endorphins.
- It may be good for your teeth because it contains theobromine, which may actually harden tooth enamel.
- It has some good nutrients like potassium, copper, magnesium, and iron.
- It may protect against sunburns.
- It may decrease coughing because it contains theobromine, which has been used as a cough suppressant.
- Drinking cocoa rich in flavonols has been shown to boost blood flow to the brain.

PART FOUR:

Eating for Your Health

CHAPTER 12

Bonus Health Benefits

When I was teaching my son to read, I had absolutely no idea that we were coming up with a method to teach reading that would benefit many others. It was a bonus benefit of our own very private struggle. The same is true of the Addicto-carb Diet. It not only benefited me in a number of unexpected ways; I have also observed astounding benefits to patients in ways that I never would have imagined: to gluten sensitive and cardiac patients, diabetics, fatigued and depressed patients, and perhaps most surprising of all—skinny people.

Along with losing weight on it, I also enjoyed some surprise benefits. For instance, being of a certain age, I had prostate problems. It was certainly not life threatening, but I can tell you that waking up every hour to urinate, night after night, is no fun. Like many patients that I see, I procrastinated in going to the doctor, and when I finally went to the urologist, he promptly put me on Proscar (finasteride). It worked slowly over a few months, but it completely cured my problem. I no longer woke at night to urinate. My sleep improved, and I was less cranky and had more energy. I was very appreciative of the urologist's recommendation.

But then a funny thing happened. Having gotten rid of almost all my diabetic medication, thanks to the Addicto-carb Diet, I decided to try dropping the Proscar just to see what would happen. I figured that I would stop for a few weeks, and if the problem started coming back, then I would simply go back on it. Well, guess what? I haven't taken any Proscar now for a number of years. I was astounded. I called Dr. Jed Kaminetsky, a renowned urologist at New York University Medical Center, to ask him if this was possible. He said he was not surprised. I called him a few months later to ask again because I was still incredulous that after a decade on Proscar, I no longer needed it. He told me again that he was not surprised. A few months later, still incredulous, I called yet again with the same query and got the same response. This time I asked him what he thought the mechanism was.

"Weight loss and diabetic control," was his simple answer. I am not sure why I was surprised.

It is well known that overweight men have higher recurrences of prostate cancer. I have often tried to get my prostate cancer patients to lose weight for exactly that reason. Also well known is that belly fat is basically an inflammatory condition. The higher the level of inflammatory compounds in the body, the more likely a man is to suffer from prostatic enlargement. But what was probably the kicker for me was that insulin levels are higher in people with belly fat, which causes the prostate to enlarge because of an increase of insulin growth factor.[1]

That made me wonder about the way I treat enlarged prostates in men with frequent urination. How many men had I put on Proscar over the years? A lot, and with tremendous success. While I always told them to lose weight, I now go out of my way to especially stress it using myself as an example. For some reason it seems easier for patients to accept if they know that it is part of my own personal journey.

Exactly how big of a problem is prostate enlargement that causes frequent urination? Very big! This is obvious by the plethora of TV commercials appealing to men with frequent urination. While the estimates vary, a conservative estimate of this problem is that around 50 percent of men approaching age fifty have it, and 75 percent of men by age eighty.[2]

Another situation with prostates comes to mind. Men who are overweight are not only more likely to get prostate cancer, but prostate cancer tends to be more aggressive in these men. So, losing weight will help you avoid getting prostate cancer, and even if you have prostate cancer, losing weight may decrease its aggressiveness.[3]

Dr. J, a prominent theologian, has been my patient for almost a quarter century. We have been through a lot together, including heart surgery and prostate cancer. He has been heavy for a long time and I have been after him for almost as long as I have known him to lose some weight. He has always said he would try but never really did. Finally he came in recently complaining about his hip. This occurred at the same time as a reemergence of his prostate cancer. Once again I was concerned, and this time I recommended the Addicto-carb Diet.

Perhaps it was the fact that the orthopedic surgeon told him he needed to lose weight before hip surgery, or the worsening of his prostate cancer, or maybe I just wore him down. Whatever the reason, he decided to go on the diet. He was overwhelmed not only by how much weight he had lost, but also the fact that it had been easy. Here's what Dr. J says about his experience:

"When Dr. Roseman told me I needed to lose weight, I told him, 'There's no hope, Doctor. I can't lose weight.' He had heard that before. So he gave me the Addictocarb Diet, and proved me wrong. In the first five weeks I lost fifteen pounds."

About six weeks later he called me again. My nurse, Nicole, told him I was with a patient. When I had a break, Nicole said to me, "Dr. J just wanted me to tell you that he has lost over twenty pounds." I can only say that his good news made *my* day. His weight loss was good for his hips and I almost fell out of my chair when I saw his PSA test had dropped dramatically, indicating that his prostate cancer had gone into remission.

The discussion of obesity and prostate cancer is important, but frankly it is just as important to note that obesity is also related to other cancers such as esophageal, pancreatic, colon, rectal, breast (after menopause), endometrial (lining of the uterus), kidney, thyroid, and gallbladder.[4]

So what is my point? My point is that the Addictocarb Diet works on a variety of levels to cure or ameliorate a range of illnesses, cancer being just one. I now go out of my way to suggest my diet to men with prostate issues; but there is more.

For example, gluten awareness is big now, as I mentioned in chapter nine. You can get gluten-free everything everywhere now, as opposed to just a few years ago when it was almost impossible to keep to a gluten-free diet. The Addictocarb Diet, by virtue of eliminating many gluten-rich foods and providing gluten-free Addictocarb Alternatives, dramatically improves the lives of people with some gluten sensitivity. If you choose to go totally gluten free on the Addictocarb Diet, you are almost there by avoiding most gluten-rich foods like bread. Also, I mention alternatives for pasta, such as quinoa pasta, and alternatives for Wasa crackerbreads, such as Natural Nectars Cracklebred. With a little vigilance to avoid hidden sources of gluten (wheat, barley, and rye) by checking ingredients in store-bought foods like meatballs, sausage, beer, and hundreds of other things—even tea—it's easy to be totally gluten free on the Addictocarb Diet.

The Addictocarb Diet is a weight loss and maintenance diet. It has worked for me and many hundreds of my patients. Yet the fact that people feel so good on the diet certainly makes me question if it is *only* because of weight loss. I don't think so. I am constantly astounded by how good my patients feel after going on the Addictocarb Diet, and it has been one of the greatest satisfactions of my life. I will not pretend that it was part of the master plan, because these salutary effects were all unintended benefits of the Addictocarb Diet, but nevertheless I am certainly happy about it, and so are my patients. But there is one patient who really surprised me.

Meryl is a fifty-five-year-old woman who has been a patient of mine for twenty-five years. She has always eaten moderately and kept herself in peak physical condition through ballroom dancing. She was in the office one day for a reason that had absolutely nothing to do with diet advice. She noticed I had lost a lot of weight and asked about my "secret."

I was surprised; she was thin, in great shape, and I knew that she ate well because we had discussed dietary issues over the years, such as glutens, organics, and antioxidants. So when I told her about the diet, and she wanted to learn more, I was happy to send her some of the chapters of *The Addictocarb Diet*. I thought it would be a great opportunity to get some feedback on the book from someone who was smart and thoughtful. In fact, her feedback threw me for a loop. Her response was so far off of what I was expecting, it was shocking.

This came up during a time when I was writing the book and giving chapters to my patients at an ever-increasing rate. People were calling me constantly for advice about the diet, or to ask if they could give it to their friends who were amazed by their weight loss. I was gratified that so many people found the diet helpful, but never once did I anticipate that a health-conscious, slim person in great physical shape would be interested in my diet. I was wrong.

Meryl told me that *The Addictocarb Diet* had changed her life. I could explain here what she told me but, when I asked her if she would write a few thoughts for the Addictocarb website, she wrote such a touching, thoughtful, and beautifully crafted piece I felt it was best to just share it with you here:

I am hooked on Dr. Roseman's Addictocarb Diet!

Dr. Roseman was surprised when I told him that, like him, I struggled with food. I am slim, have danced all my life, and do not appear to have food issues. But I come from a family of overeaters who like to snack. Many are overweight, and the ones who are not work hard to keep off the pounds.

Dr. Roseman's Addictocarb Diet has made my own challenge with food easier, because it offers a framework I can follow. I know bread, potatoes, and processed sweets will set up cravings, so I simply avoid them. So far, it has been an easy and painless transition, and the rewards have come quickly.

Gone are my desires for crackers, granola bars, and my daily oatmeal breakfast. My go-to snacks are now protein Shakes, fruit, nuts, and hot quinoa in the morning. The protein Shake is key: It fills me up and tastes delicious!

It's been three months since I started the Addictocarb Diet. My jeans are looser and the visceral fat that appeared at menopause, and with which I have been trying to make peace, is slowly melting away.

—Meryl Weiss

The Addictocarb Diet works on many levels to improve health. Eating all the berries and other fruits in the Shakes is good for a variety of maladies, perhaps related to all those antioxidants in them or their anti-inflammatory properties. The diet is good for middle-aged women who want to lose their "middle-age spare tire" and for men with prostate issues. It is good for people with gluten sensitivity. It is certainly good for diabetics. It can also work for the lactose intolerant.

In short, while the Addictocarb Diet it is a great weight loss diet, the bonus health benefits of the diet continue to surprise and amaze me.

CHAPTER 13

Diabetes: Prevent It—
Treat It—Beat It

When it comes to diabetes, I unfortunately speak from personal experience. More than ten years ago, my doctor diagnosed me with diabetes. For the next year I was put on several oral diabetic medications with varying degrees of success. Each one worked a little, yet my diabetes kept getting worse, so the next step was seeing an endocrinologist. He, too, tried varying my oral medications for a few months, again with only minimal success, until that fateful day when he handed me a prescription for injectable diabetes medicine.

I was crushed, and could hardly believe it. I did not want to give myself insulin injections, but I started using them—first exenatide, then insulin. I hated them. I knew that the way to treat diabetes was with diet and exercise,[1] and I already swam a mile a day and walked three miles. Clearly the exercise was not working, so that left one suspect—my diet. I finally accepted the reality: The only way for me to treat my diabetes was to lose weight. What was I going to do?

I knew I needed to lose *at least* thirty pounds, and I realized that I was addicted to food, so I set out to construct a diet by digesting the medical literature on behavioral addiction. The Addictocarb Diet is what came out of that research. I was as surprised as anyone when I ended up losing almost sixty pounds, but as my health improved, I also have stopped taking almost all medication for diabetes.

Diabetes is the most significant medical problem confronting the American population today, with more than 100 million diabetics and prediabetics. Let's just look at the raw numbers from the American Diabetes Association: 25.8 million children and adults in the United States—8.3 percent of the population—have diabetes, and 79 million people are prediabetic,[2] which, as far as I am concerned, is exactly the same thing as having diabetes.

Why is it such a big deal? Adults with diabetes have heart disease death rates and risk of stroke two to four times higher than adults without diabetes. Diabetes is the leading cause of kidney failure and of new cases of blindness among adults. Sixty to 70 percent of diabetics have nervous system damage. It is a major cause of amputations, accounting for more than 60 percent of nontraumatic lower-limb amputations. Prior to starting the Addictocarb Diet to manage my own diabetes, I had to face the possibility of losing some of my toes, barely avoiding it with painful daily intramuscular injections for over a month.

To sum up, diabetes is important because it causes painful, debilitating diseases that lead to death, which can all be avoided and even cured by early diagnosis and proper treatment—and by proper treatment in this context, I mean the Addictocarb Diet coupled with exercise.

What exactly is diabetes? Simplified, diabetes is a disease related to sugar in the blood and the pancreatic hormone insulin, which processes the sugar (glucose) in the bloodstream, transporting it out of the blood to areas where sugar is needed. This is very important because sugar is a source of energy for your muscles, tissues, and brain. Having too little insulin causes too much sugar to accumulate in the blood, which damages the blood vessels. Damaged blood vessels cause serious end organ damage, like heart attacks, kidney failure, blindness, amputations, and other terrible things.

There are two types of diabetes, type 1 and type 2. Type 1 generally occurs in younger people who have no insulin, and type 2 is usually found in older people who just run out of insulin over a period of time. The main cause of type 2 diabetes is obesity. When I first went into practice, the only people I saw with type 2 diabetes were people older than sixty. Over the past decade, however, I started seeing more and younger people, in their thirties and forties, coming in with type 2 diabetes. Many articles have noted that this is a common trend in America.[3] The *Journal of the American Medical Association* recently reported that there has been a staggering increase in type 2 diabetes in children less than nineteen years of age,[4] and this used to be referred to as *adult* onset diabetes. Not only is this shocking, but it is also a very bad prognostic sign for society in general, with some experts predicting that by 2050, half of the United States population will have some type of diabetes.

How does this happen? Insulin is manufactured in the pancreas, an organ located in the abdomen behind the stomach and attached to the small intestine and spleen. Inside the pancreas there are small clusters of things called beta cells that produce insulin. In people who do not have diabetes, sugar in the blood stimulates the production of insulin in the beta cells. Beta cells constantly monitor blood sugar levels and deliver the required amount of insulin to the bloodstream, where it transports the sugar into the various cells in the body. In a normal person this usually keeps the blood sugar levels between 60 and 120 mg/dL and another key indicator, hemoglobin A1c (HbA1c, or A1c for short), under 5.7.

A convenient way to think about it is to imagine the pancreas as an ATM for insulin. Children think that money comes from ATM machines. They do not understand that you can only take out money if you have money in the bank, and if you use it up too fast then you will not have any left. The same is true of insulin. When the body needs insulin, it takes some out of the pancreatic ATM. There are things that make you use up more insulin so that you run out faster. There are also things that allow you to use less insulin so that you run out more slowly. Things that make you use up more insulin faster are Addictocarbs. Things that allow you to use less insulin are exercise, certain medications, and the Addictocarb Diet. Some medications allow the insulin you do have to be used more efficiently, and some drugs manage to squeeze more insulin out of the pancreas. Eventually many people with type 2 diabetes end up in the same boat with type 1 diabetics; they just do not have enough insulin, and they are forced to obtain it through injections.

Addictocarbs are terrible for you in two relevant ways. First, their impact on the brain's addiction center makes it hard for you to lose weight and keep it off. Second, all Addictocarbs are high-glycemic foods, though not all high-glycemic foods are Addictocarbs. The glycemic index is essentially a measure of how rapidly and how much insulin is caused to pour into your bloodstream by eating certain foods. Bread, potatoes, sugary things, and the other Addictocarbs in general have a very high glycemic index.

Going back to our ATM analogy, Addictocarbs cause you to run out of insulin faster. The ATM warns you that you are out of money with a painless message on a screen. The pancreas lets you know you have run out of insulin by causing diabetes, which leads to blindness, amputations, kidney failure, heart attacks, and strokes.

The ways you know you are in the throes of diabetes are the classic three Ps: polyuria (the need to urinate frequently), polydipsia (increased thirst and fluid intake), and polyphagia (increased appetite). But there are other early warning signs, such as feeling tired and sluggish after eating, craving carbs more than usual, being generally overweight, and high blood pressure, which may result from weight gain and increasing girth.

In fact, one way that has been accepted for years to measure the healthy weight of an individual is the BMI, which may actually give misleading results. A better tool is something called the ABSI, which is a measure of weight that takes into account your girth (waist size). This calculator was developed at The City College of New York, and is the best indicator of whether you are of a healthy weight.[5] Another calculator with a better interface can be found at http://www.absi-calculator.com.

The reason this is so important is that girth relates to internal (visceral) fat deposition, the fat inside your body. Just because you have flabby arms does not mean you will get diabetes, but if your girth or belt size is elevated, that is a sign that you have a lot of internal fat deposition, which puts you at high risk for diabetes. The proper way to measure your girth is to measure as you would for a belt (at the level of the iliac crest, the bone that sticks out at the level of your waist).

How do you diagnose diabetes? According to the ADA, a number of tests can be used, the most useful of which is A1c. This blood test measures your average blood sugar for the previous three months. The advantages of being diagnosed this way are that you don't have to fast or drink anything. The values are:[6]

Result	A1c Level
Normal	less than 5.7%
Prediabetes	5.7% to 6.4%
Diabetes	6.5% or higher

The biggest problem with the A1c test is that not enough doctors use it. A lot of them still just check a regular blood sugar level, which will miss a lot of early-stage diabetics. This is important because if you discover diabetes early, you will have plenty of time to forestall and even cure the disease. I recommend that anytime you get a physical from your doctor, or have your blood drawn for any reason, make sure to ask for an A1c test.

If you have an A1c of over 6.5 percent, you have diabetes, and if your result is between 5.7 and 6.4 percent, this indicates prediabetes, which means you will probably develop diabetes unless you take steps to avoid it. Frankly, I have no idea why they even use the term "prediabetes." When you conceive, do they refer to you as being pre-pregnant? No. The same thing is true for diabetes. It is a bogus diagnostic category. Either you have diabetes or you don't. It could be a mild case or a severe, life-threatening case. When I speak to my "prediabetic" patients I explain to them that as far as I am concerned, they have diabetes because they have to do the exact same things to treat prediabetes as diabetes. And then I explain the Addictocarb Diet to them.

The important thing to understand about prediabetes, early diabetes, or even regular type 2 diabetes, is that it is usually caused by obesity. If you lose weight and stick to the Addictocarb Diet, the disease will get better. In my case, my A1c was 9.4, which by anyone's definition is diabetes. Through nothing more than going on the Addictocarb Diet, my last A1c at my cardiologist was 5.7. My reaction when he called to tell me was that it had to be a mistake. Even though I have seen this in my own patients, as a patient myself, I was still stunned when he told me. How could l have possibly fallen from a high of 9.4 to 5.7, especially since I had stopped taking almost all my diabetes medications? The answer is the Addictocarb Diet.

My story accentuates the importance of early diagnosis. If you catch diabetes early, you can sometimes cure it, forestall it, or at the very least mitigate its ravages. Even the American Diabetes Association says that if you have prediabetes, you will not *necessarily* develop type 2 diabetes. For some people with prediabetes, early treatment can actually return blood sugar levels to the normal range. Research shows that you can lower your risk for type 2 diabetes by 58 percent simply by losing 7 percent of your body weight (about fourteen pounds if you weigh 200 pounds) and exercising moderately (such as brisk walking) for thirty minutes a day, five days a week.

I want to be very clear here: If you have early diabetes (prediabetes) and you go on the Addictocarb Diet, you will forestall getting diabetes and may even cure it. That is exactly what happened to me and many of my patients. My blood sugar went from the 300s to the low 100s, and my A1c from 9.4 to 5.7. I have had patients with early diabetes who have gone on the Addictocarb Diet and seen their A1c return to completely normal. The Addictocarb Diet can reduce A1c levels quickly, but that's not the only reason for starting it. The Addictocarb Diet will help you keep the weight off permanently, and thus comes as close to a natural cure for diabetes as you can get.

PART FIVE:

The Addictocarb Diet Recipes and Menus

Before getting into the recipes themselves, here are my general cooking and eating tips.

- In general for any given food, the less processed it is the better.
- For every single recipe that calls for butter, margarine, or cooking spray, I use Smart Balance or Benecol, which are far healthier and help lower cholesterol to boot.
- For every single recipe that calls for sugar, I use my sweeteners recipes on page 130.
- In general, anytime a recipe calls for eggs, I use Eggbeaters® because it has no cholesterol and very few calories. If you are going to use eggs, try to use omega-3 eggs, organic if possible.
- Flaxseed meal is high in fiber and omega-3, which help lower cholesterol. It is good for digestive health and constipation, and also for cancer, heart disease, diabetes, and inflammation, among other things. So anytime you can put flaxseed meal in any recipe, do it. Pancakes, soup, burgers, and kasha varnishkes are good options. I strongly suggest ground to whole seeds and keep refrigerated.
- When using milk, try to use only organic and preferably skim milk or nut and soy milks.
- Try to buy organic apples, pears, and peaches, or at least wash them carefully before eating because of pesticides.
- Anytime there is a chance to use a low-sodium anything, such as stock or even vegetable juice, do it.
- For every single recipe that uses meat (beef, pork, and veal), eat three or more strawberries, which you can either mix in with the dish or eat straight up. You can read the whole boxed section about berries and meat on page 55.

A NOTE ON SWEETENERS

Sometimes you need something to sweeten up a recipe, such as oatmeal, which, after all, leaves something to be desired in the taste department. How are you going to sweeten it? I have spent hours and hours in the kitchen testing various sweeteners against changes in my blood sugar and this is what I have come up with.

These recipes will hold for just about any fruit, like peaches and pears, but I have found that bananas and apples seem to work best. If you have any other suggestions, please send them to me on my website at http://www.Addictocarb.com.

Apple: This can be done in either a blender or food processor, but the best way to do this is with something like the NutriBullet, which is relatively inexpensive, has other uses, and is easy to clean. The process is actually quite simple. You simply cut up an apple (I prefer McIntosh for this) into one-inch pieces, leaving the peel on if organic, and removing the peel if not, and toss the pieces in the NutriBullet or processor. Process for about thirty seconds, and you essentially have a finely pureed applesauce. If you use a food processor it will not be as fine, but it will work just as well. Simply use this as a sweetener. It is delicious.

Banana: Mash a banana very smooth with an avocado or potato masher, or a fork, and use it as a sweetener. Once again, absolutely delicious.

CHAPTER 14

Addictocarb Alternative
Recipes for Bread

use Wasa Crisp'n Light Crackerbreads as a bread alternative for just about anything that I'd use bread for. Cut up,
it becomes croutons in a salad; dipped in olive oil, it is the
perfect surrogate for a bread basket; I even use it to make desserts. I also use it to make all different kinds of sandwiches,
some as simple as peanut butter and banana, others slightly
more complex.

There are other creative bread alternatives, such as lettuce
leaf sandwiches and other low-carb and even gluten-free crackers on the market that could be used instead of the Wasa brand,
but this is my preference after a decade of experience both
personally and with almost a thousand patients. If you discover
other alternatives, I would love to hear about them. Please send
them in to my website, http://www.Addictocarb.com.

The basil, ham, and cheese sandwich is my personal favorite, so I will start with that.

THE BASIL, HAM, AND CHEESE SANDWICH

The great thing about this sandwich is that it tastes good
and has protein, which fills me up. It does not raise my blood

sugar, and it fits perfectly into my diet so that I can eat it and lose weight or just stay thin.

Yield: 1 sandwich

Ingredients:

- 2 thin slices ham
- 2 thin slices cheddar cheese (I prefer extra sharp)
- mustard to taste (I prefer Dijon, but any mustard will do— except sweetened mustards)
- 2 large leaves fresh basil
- 2 leaves lettuce
- 2 slices Wasa Crisp'n Light Crackerbreads

Directions:

1. Stack the ingredients on the crackerbreads just like you would a regular sandwich and serve.

One of the secrets of a great sandwich is fresh basil, which can easily be purchased year round. Besides adding to the taste, the aroma just slays me. Occasionally, I soak the basil in olive oil. I hope you enjoy it guilt free.

MY FAVORITE ROAST BEEF SANDWICH

This sandwich was one of my all-time favorites on bread. I am actually surprised at how well it holds up using the Wasa crackers. It meets all the requirements for my diet. It gives you protein to satiate your hunger, a modest amount of carbs, and an interesting mix of ingredients. When I eat this sandwich, I do it totally guilt free. It does not raise my blood sugar, and I do not feel even remotely deprived. Sometimes my skinny wife even says, "Hey, I'll have one of those, too."

Yield: 1 sandwich

Ingredients:
- 2 slices Wasa Crisp'n Light Crackerbreads
- plain cream cheese
- ½ teaspoon horseradish (white or red)
- 2–3 thin slices roast beef

Directions:
1. Smear the cream cheese on one crackerbread, then smear it with the horseradish.
2. Put the roast beef on the other slice of crackerbread, join the two halves, and you've got yourself a really easy and delicious sandwich.

In some places you can actually buy horseradish cream cheese, which makes it a lot easier.

CELERY DILL TUNA SANDWICH

I love tuna salad, and I am crazy about dill, onions, and mayo. I used to think it had to be eaten on bread. I will not deny that is good, but frankly so is this. I either eat it off a plate or with the Wasa crackerbreads to take the place of bread.

Yield: 4 sandwiches

Ingredients:
- 1 can tuna
- 2 tablespoons mayonnaise
- ⅛ cup diced onion
- ¼ cup diced celery
- 2 tablespoons fresh dill, finely minced
- ½ teaspoon Dijon mustard

- pinch table salt
- 8 slices Wasa Crisp'n Light Crackerbreads
- 4 slices muenster or other cheese (optional)

Directions:

1. In a bowl, mash up the tuna to your preference (I like it fine and my wife likes it chunky), making sure to separate the pieces.
2. Add the mayo and mix well.
3. Add the onion, celery, dill, mustard, and salt, and mix well.
4. If using muenster, place a slice on a piece of crackerbread and put the tuna salad on top. Top it off with another slice of crackerbread. Repeat for the remaining sandwiches and serve.

PEANUT BUTTER AND RASPBERRIES SANDWICH

Okay, I am not fooling anyone here. This is a variation of peanut butter and jelly, one of the all-time greats of sandwichdom. It is certainly one of my favorites, though in truth it is more like a dessert than a lunch sandwich, but it works either way. It appeals to me for a number of reasons, not the least of which is that my drive to make beautiful food and need to organize is allowed to flourish, as I neatly arrange and fix the raspberries on the bed of luscious, rich peanut butter. This is one sandwich I actually enjoy making more than eating, although I do truly love to eat it. When I am in a really indulgent mood, I add thin slices of banana. Peanut butter, raspberries, and banana—it does not get any better than that.

Once again, it meets all the requirements of the diet. It provides protein for satiety, and the crackerbreads and raspberries for the carbs. It is *sort* of like eating peanut butter and jelly, but better, because it has the fruit flavor we love in jelly without all that sugar.

Yield: 1 sandwich

Ingredients:
- 2 slices Wasa Crisp'n Light Crackerbreads
- peanut butter (I prefer super chunky or homemade in the blender)
- about 10 or 12 fresh raspberries
- ½ banana (optional)

Directions:
1. Smear the crackerbreads with desired amount of peanut butter.
2. Neatly arrange the raspberries on the beds of peanut butter. I always compete with myself to see how many I can get on the crackerbread. I usually do it in two neat rows, though I have been known to add an entire third row, in which case I may have to cut the raspberries in half in order to get them to fit. When I am in a really indulgent mood, I add the optional banana.
3. I usually serve the sandwich open faced, but I occasionally join the two slices of crackerbread to make it feel more like a sandwich.

JOSHUA'S CHOPPED AVOCADO–BURGER SALAD

I am not sure that this should really be included with the bread alternative recipes because it is really a salad. On the other hand, the Wasa Crisp'n Light Crackerbreads make stupendous croutons, and, after all, what is a salad without croutons?

My son Joshua tends to have a weight problem. He lost twenty pounds on the Addictocarb Diet and has kept it off. He also fancies himself a serious chef. Nevertheless, when I first saw him make this, I was flabbergasted. My gastronomic sense was offended as I watched him chop everything up and toss it in a bowl. However, his recipe met all of the requisites of the Addictocarb Diet. He did not want to eat the hamburger on a bun, and he did not want to eat a salad without croutons. Combining them made sense.

It was my wife who first said, "I'll try some of that." Seeing that my wife and son were both enjoying the salad, I just had to taste it, too. I was hooked after the first bite. This is a great salad, and the croutons perfectly top it off. I have recommended it to my patients and they also seem to love it.

Yield: 1 serving as a full meal, 4 servings as a side dish

Ingredients:
- 1 cooked hamburger patty, chopped
- 3 large leaves lettuce, chopped into about 1-inch pieces
- 1 avocado, chopped into ½-inch cubes
- 1 tomato, chopped into ½-inch cubes
- ½ onion, roughly chopped
- 2–3 tablespoons fresh cilantro, minced
- 2 Wasa Crisp'n Light Crackerbreads, cut up into croutons
- hot sauce (optional)

Directions:
1. In a large salad bowl, toss together all the ingredients. Serve.

My son eats this salad (and everything else) with hot sauce and lots of people seem to like it, so I included it here. When I make this salad for myself, I prefer a simple oil and vinegar dressing, using three parts oil to one part vinegar. You can also use any commercially prepared dressing. Just check to make sure it does not have any added sugar or high fructose corn syrup.

CAULIFLOWER PIZZA

One day while chopping up and processing cauliflower to make Wendy's Mashed Unpotato (page 142), I had an idea: Why not just fry the stuff in the pan and see how it tastes? Soon enough I found out that if something seems too good to be true it probably is. Everything fell apart in the pan.

After seeking some counsel from my nurse, Nicole, who had actually made cauliflower pizzas, and after multiple failed attempts, including trying to make it healthier by baking instead of frying, I finally came up with a recipe that works. I added some Italian seasonings and binding agents. Nothing brilliant here; it is remarkably similar to eating pizza, but this recipe definitely does not contain Addictocarbs—and it is really good.

Yield: four 6-inch pizzas

Ingredients:
- 1 head cauliflower
- 1 clove garlic, minced
- 2 tablespoons minced fresh basil, divided
- 2 cups shredded mozzarella cheese, divided
- ⅛ teaspoon dried oregano
- 1 large egg, beaten
- 4–6 tablespoons tomato sauce (page 149 or use store-bought)
- 2 tablespoons grated parmesan cheese

Directions:
1. Preheat the oven to 450°F.
2. Chop up the cauliflower into small pieces and cook until soft. You can microwave the pieces in 3 tablespoons of water for 15–20 minutes, steam them, or boil them.
3. Allow the cauliflower to cool for about 10 minutes and then chop it up into even smaller pieces. Drop the cauliflower

slowly into a food processor and process until smooth. Set aside in a bowl.

4. Place the cauliflower in cheesecloth, a towel, or even a paper towel and squeeze out as much moisture as possible.

5. Put the garlic and 1 tablespoon of basil in the food processor and mince for 10 seconds.

6. Put 2 cups of the processed cauliflower in a bowl and set aside remainder to use in another recipe. Add 1 ½ cups of shredded mozzarella, the oregano, the processed garlic and basil, and the beaten egg and mix it well with a fork.

7. Divide the mixture into four parts and form each part into a ball. Place each ball on a lightly greased baking sheet or parchment paper and pat them down until flat, making sure that you crimp each pizza around the outside so that you get a nice crust that is slightly elevated around the edge.

8. Bake for 15–18 minutes until the crusts are slightly crispy around the edges.

9. Remove from the oven and spoon tomato sauce on top of each. Then sprinkle with remaining ½ cup of mozzarella and parmesan cheese and top off with remaining tablespoon of basil.

10. Put the pizzas back in the oven for another 5 minutes so that the cheese on top melts, then remove and let cool for 5 minutes before serving.

BACON CHEDDAR BURGERS

This may seem like another strange recipe for the bread alternative section, but it can be eaten sandwiched between two large lettuce leaves or even on a crackerbread. I am not, by any stretch of the imagination, promoting this as a *healthy* recipe, because of its high fat content, but nevertheless it fits the diet. It is a guilty pleasure that some people simply cannot give up, though perhaps it is something you should discuss with your doctor.

Yield: 4 hamburgers

Ingredients:

- 1 pound hamburger meat
- ½ cup shredded cheddar cheese
- 4 slices bacon, diced
- 8 large lettuce leaves (optional)

Directions:

1. In a large bowl, knead together the hamburger, cheese, and bacon. Form mixture into four patties.
2. Pan-fry the patties, enjoying the guilty pleasure of the bacon aroma wafting through the house.
3. If you wish, you can serve the patties sandwiched between two large lettuce leaves and add any of your preferred Addictocarb-free burger toppings.

CHAPTER 15

Addictocarb Alternative Recipes for Potatoes

There are not a lot of alternatives to potatoes. The best alternative in my mind is simply to substitute sweet potatoes for regular. This works quite well for things like French fries (better baked, not fried) and baked potatoes. I wrote in chapter six about the sweet potato revolution in this country. It has become so much easier to find them in the frozen food sections in supermarkets.

JODIE'S ROASTED SWEET POTATOES AND PECANS

Jodie is famous in my office for always delighting us with home-cooked foods. When I asked her for a sweet potato recipe, she sent this over immediately. It is great.

Yield: 4 servings

Ingredients:
- 4 medium sweet potatoes, peeled and sliced into ¾-inch discs
- ¼ cup vegetable oil
- 1 teaspoon ground ginger
- ½ teaspoon ground cinnamon

- ¼ teaspoon ground cardamom
- ¼ teaspoon garlic powder
- table salt and black pepper, to taste
- ⅓ cup chopped pecans
- 2 tablespoons low-calorie maple pancake syrup

Directions:

1. Preheat the oven to 400°F.
2. Put the sweet potato discs into a bowl and drizzle with the vegetable oil, taking care to coat all the pieces.
3. In another bowl, combine the spices and pecans and mix.
4. Add the pancake syrup and spice mixture to the bowl with the sweet potato and mix.
5. Spray a rimmed cookie sheet with a neutral cooking spray and arrange the potato discs in a single layer.
6. Place the potato discs in the oven for 10 minutes or until they brown, then flip with a spatula and cook until the other side is browned or caramelized and fork tender.
7. Remove from oven and serve while still warm.

WENDY'S MASHED UNPOTATO

This is one of the ways that some people deal with not being able to eat potatoes: by *not using* potatoes and trying to re-create the experience with more healthy fare. It may not be perfect, but lots of people seem to like it. It is a fascinating take on mashed potatoes and fits in perfectly with the diet. No Addictocarbs here.

Yield: 4 servings (as a side)

Ingredients:

- 1 head cauliflower
- 1 14-ounce can artichoke hearts, stored in water
- 1–2 garlic cloves, minced (optional)
- table salt to taste

- pinch coarse black pepper
- garlic powder to taste (optional)

Directions:

1. Cook the head of cauliflower until soft by either steaming or microwaving it. Chop it into small pieces.
2. Put the cauliflower, artichokes, garlic (if using), salt, and pepper in a blender and puree to the consistency of mashed potatoes.
3. Transfer mixture to a pan. Warm on the stove, and add garlic powder if desired. Serve.

NICOLE'S SWEET POTATO FRIES WITH GARLIC AIOLI

Nicole, my nurse, likes to eat. She also likes to stay thin and eat healthy. She hits on all cylinders with this recipe.

Yield: 4 servings

Ingredients:

- 1 large sweet potato
- olive oil, to coat

Sprinkle Mixture #1

- ¼ tablespoon table salt
- ¼ tablespoon black pepper
- ½ tablespoon garlic salt
- ¼ teaspoon paprika

Sprinkle Mixture #2

- 2 tablespoons chopped fresh parsley
- 1 tablespoon grated parmesan cheese

Garlic Aioli Dipping Sauce

- 1–2 cloves garlic, finely minced
- ¼ cup mayonnaise
- 3 teaspoons lemon juice, more or less to taste

- black pepper, to taste
- table salt, to taste

Directions:

1. Preheat the oven to 450°F.
2. Peel and slice the sweet potato into ½-inch-thick fries and toss them in enough olive oil to coat.
3. Sprinkle potatoes with mixture #1 and spread them evenly across parchment paper on a baking sheet.
4. Bake for 12 minutes, turning once at the halfway point.
5. Remove fries and sprinkle with mixture #2. Toss to coat evenly.
6. Combine all the ingredients for the garlic aioli and serve with the fries as a dipping sauce.

NICOLE'S SWEET POTATO LATKES

Potato latkes are delicious and celebratory. They are also fattening and made of Addictocarbs like potatoes and flour. *This* latke recipe, however, is different. Nicole made them for me and they were great. To my amazement, they actually *lowered* my blood sugar.

Nicole simply substituted the potatoes with an Addictocarb Alternative, sweet potatoes, which have a lower glycemic index and fewer calories and cause fewer cravings. Sweet potatoes are also good for those with diabetes.

In this recipe, we also use a minimal amount of an Addictocarb Accommodation in the whole wheat flour. It is always best to bake these, but you can fry them if you must.

Yield: 4 servings

Ingredients:

- 1 medium sweet potato, shredded
- 1 medium onion, finely chopped

- 2 tablespoons whole wheat flour
- ¼ teaspoon kosher salt
- black pepper, to taste
- 1 egg, slightly beaten
- applesauce (page 177, optional)
- sour cream (optional)

Directions:

1. In a large bowl, mix together all of the ingredients except for the applesauce and sour cream.
2. *If baking*: Preheat the oven to 400°F. Generously grease a cookie sheet. Drop the sweet potato mixture by teaspoonfuls onto cookie sheet and flatten them slightly. Bake for 12–15 minutes, turning once, until golden brown.
3. *If frying*: In 12-inch skillet, heat ¼ cup of vegetable oil over medium-high heat. Drop sweet potato mixture by teaspoonfuls into skillet and flatten them slightly. Cook for 4–5 minutes, turning once, until golden brown. Drain the cooked latkes of extra oil on paper towels.
4. Serve with applesauce or sour cream.

CHAPTER 16

Addictocarb Alternative Recipes for Pasta

In terms of pasta alternatives there are a few. You can substitute the Dreamfields pasta in any recipe with quinoa pasta, tofu pasta, and Jerusalem artichoke pasta. These will all work, but to my taste, Dreamfields is the best alternative. In chapter six, I explained in detail that Dreamfields pasta has a low glycemic index as a result of fewer absorbed carbs and is therefore less fattening and causes less intense cravings. Jerusalem artichoke pasta supposedly works similarly. Whole wheat pasta is like brown rice, and it is better for you than regular pasta, but it is still made of an Addictocarb and may raise blood sugar and cause cravings. Like brown rice, it is an Accommodation in that it is far better than eating regular pasta, but not as good as an alternative like Dreamfields.

GARLIC FRIED SPAGHETTI

The flour-pasta version of this has been one of my favorite foods of all time. It is easy to prepare and tastes great, and the kids were always happy to have it. Unfortunately, I found that once I started eating the flour version, I could not stop. I do not have that problem now that I substitute Dreamfields pasta.

Yield: 2–4 servings

Ingredients:

- 1 pound Dreamfields spaghetti
- ⅓ cup olive oil (preferably extra virgin)
- 4 cloves garlic, minced

Directions:

1. Put the spaghetti into 6 quarts of boiling water and cook until al dente.
2. While the spaghetti is cooking, add the olive oil to a large heated sauté pan along with the minced garlic and cook it on low heat until the garlic just starts to brown.
3. Remove the spaghetti from the water and strain. Add it to the sauté pan and fry it for a few moments, toss it, then fry for another few moments. Repeat until all of the spaghetti has been coated and fried in the oil.

ALEX'S BOLOGNESE SAUCE

This sauce is very different from my own Plain and Easy Tomato Sauce (page 149) and lends itself better to pasta. The recipe was given to me by a patient who throws wonderful Sunday dinners at her house. I tasted this sauce at one such dinner and, since it fits the Addictocarb lifestyle, I immediately begged her for the recipe. She was more than gracious in going over it with me in detail. It fills the house with an intense aroma that I feel evokes thoughts of a wonderful family dinner.

Yield: 8 servings

Ingredients:

- 1 sprig parsley
- 1 medium onion, diced

- 1 stalk celery, diced
- 1 medium carrot, diced
- 2 cloves garlic, minced
- 3 tablespoons olive oil
- 2 tablespoons butter
- 1 slice prosciutto, coarsely chopped
- 1 pound mixture of ground beef, pork, and veal
- pinch dried sage
- kosher salt and black pepper, to taste
- ¼ cup dry white wine
- 3 tablespoons tomato paste
- 1 8-ounce can tomato sauce
- 2 cups chicken or beef stock
- ½ cup heavy cream

Directions:

1. Add prosciutto, parsley, and all vegetables together in a food processor and chop to a very fine mixture.
2. In a saucepan, heat oil and butter. Add the chopped prosciutto and vegetable mixture and cook, stirring until completely wilted and soft.
3. Add ground meat and cook until brown. Stir often and break up lumps of meat while cooking.
4. Add sage, salt, and pepper. Pour in wine and cook, uncovered, until wine evaporates.
5. Add tomato paste and tomato sauce. Cook mixture until well blended.
6. Add stock and mix well. Cover and bring to a boil. Reduce heat and let simmer covered for about 1 hour.
7. Remove from heat. Add the heavy cream and stir.

PLAIN AND EASY TOMATO SAUCE

While I love my bolognese sauce (page 151) and Alex's (page 148), I also love just a basic tomato sauce—nothing but tomatoes, vegetables, and herbs. I also appreciate that some people prefer a plant-based diet, and this sauce is perfect for that. This sauce is nothing special, but I always enjoy it. The aroma slays me, and it is especially easy to make. I usually just throw everything into the food processor, although the ingredients can just as easily, and perhaps more enjoyably, be hand diced and then added into the sauté pan. It is packed with antioxidants and is a perfect Addictocarb-free food. I often keep some in the fridge for other recipes, like Cauliflower Pizza (page 137).

Yield: 4–6 servings

Ingredients:
- 1 large carrot, diced
- 1 large stalk celery, diced
- 3–4 sprigs parsley, diced
- 5 fresh basil leaves, chopped
- 1 onion, diced
- 2 cloves garlic, minced
- ½ cup olive oil
- 2 28-ounce cans peeled Italian tomatoes (preferably San Marzano)

Directions:
1. Throw the carrot, celery, parsley, basil, onion, and garlic in the food processor and process until it reaches a smooth texture, about 30 seconds. Depending on the size of your food processor you may need to process the ingredients in shifts and mix together at the end. Alternately, you can hand-dice everything, which is more fun and very aromatic.
2. Put the olive oil in a pan, add the vegetable mixture, and sauté for 3–4 minutes. Then toss in the tomatoes, including the juices from the can, and simmer for 10–15 minutes.

MY PERSONAL BOLOGNESE SAUCE

The great thing about this bolognese sauce is the way it fits into the Addictocarb lifestyle. The way that I use it most often is as a type of chili; I just eat the sauce like stew because it is filling, nutritious, and Addictocarb free. My wife prefers it with pasta, which works for her. It can be served with Addictocarb Alternatives like Dreamfields pasta or quinoa pasta, or with whole wheat pasta, an Addictocarb Accommodation. Whatever way you eat it, it is a healthy recipe and will help keep you slim.

Yield: 8 servings

Ingredients:
- 1 pound sausage meat, removed from casings and diced
- 2 pounds ground beef, pork, and veal mixture
- ½ cup olive oil
- 2 tablespoons butter
- 2 cups diced celery
- 2 cups diced carrot
- 2 cups diced onion
- 2 tablespoons chopped fresh parsley
- ⅛ teaspoon black pepper
- 1–2 teaspoons table salt (optional)
- 3–4 cloves diced garlic
- 4 28-ounce cans Italian peeled tomatoes (preferably San Marzano)
- 2 tablespoons chopped fresh basil
- 1 bay leaf
- ⅛ teaspoon chili or red pepper flakes
- 2 tablespoons Marsala wine or good drinking sherry

Directions:
1. Sauté the sausage in a pan, making sure to brown it on all sides. While cooking, break it up into the smallest pieces you can. After you finish, set it aside.

2. In the same pan, sauté the ground beef, pork, and veal mixture and set aside.
3. Put the olive oil and butter in large pot with the celery, carrot, onion, parsley, pepper, salt if using, and garlic. Sauté for about 3–5 minutes until the vegetables are soft, making sure not to burn the onion.
4. Add the tomatoes and their juice, basil, bay leaf, chili or red pepper flakes, and wine. Bring to a boil, then turn down the heat to low so that it is gently boiling and cook uncovered for about 1 ½ hours.
5. Add in all the meat and cook for another ½ hour.

The longer you let this sauce sit the better; it will be even better the next day. The problem is that it smells so good that it is almost impossible to wait.

CHAPTER 17

Addictocarb Alternative Recipes for Rice

I use three alternatives to rice, one of them being less of an alternative and more of a compromise. Kasha and quinoa are actually rice alternatives that satisfy all the tenets of the Addictocarb Diet. They are high in protein for satiety, they raise blood sugar only minimally, and they do not cause cravings.

But if you absolutely, positively must have rice, then brown rice is an Addictocarb Accommodation, and it can be used in any of these recipes. Brown rice is still an Addictocarb because it is basically white rice without the fiber. Nevertheless, it is far better for you than white rice, which is just flat out terrible for you.

KASHA VARNISHKES

Kasha is a suitable substitute for rice. You can use it to make a pilaf or put it into soups. It is great with Chinese food, stir-fried anything, or as a side dish topped with sauce. It also serves nicely as a bed for any entrée, including meat or vegetables.

Though kasha can be eaten as a simple porridge, the secret to making it as a rice substitute is eggs. Egg albumin seals the uncooked kasha with a binding that helps the kernels remain separate and keep their shapes.

Kasha varnishkes is a recipe that I loved as a child, and is a staple in many Russian households. "Varnishkes" is Russian for dumplings, but it is rarely prepared this way anymore. Nowadays, it's often combined with some type of noodles. I watched my grandmother and my mother prepare it, and I taught my son to do it the same way. He loves it. It is fun and easy and tastes great.

Yield: 2–4 servings

Ingredients:

- 1 egg
- 1 cup dry kasha
- 2 tablespoons butter, melted
- 2 cups hot chicken stock
- kosher salt and black pepper, to taste
- ½–1 pound dry Dreamfields pasta (see Tips)
- 1 large onion, thinly sliced (optional)
- 3 tablespoons Smart Balance buttery spread *light* (or Benecol)

1. Beat the egg and mix it thoroughly with the dry kasha.
2. Put the egg-kasha mixture in a skillet or saucepan on low heat and stir it constantly for about 2 minutes until the egg has dried and the kernels are separated.
3. Combine the melted butter with the hot chicken stock and add the mixture to the same pan. Let it simmer, covered, for about 7–10 minutes until the kasha kernels are soft.
4. Add salt and pepper to taste.
5. Put the Dreamfields pasta into 6 quarts of boiling water and cook until al dente, about 5–7 minutes. Mix kasha with cooked pasta.

6. If desired, sauté the sliced onion in Smart Balance or Benecol, mixing occasionally until browned. Mix with kasha varnishkes or serve on the side.

- *My mother used to add bowtie pasta. This is an Addictocarb and you cannot have it, but you can use Dreamfields pasta. Unfortunately, Dreamfields does not make bowties, but rotini, penne, or elbow macaroni works just as well.*
- *The amount of pasta you add depends on your taste, but I usually use ½ pound. My son likes more pasta; my wife likes less.*
- *My son likes his kasha varnishkes mixed with the sautéed onions. Personally I prefer to place them on the table so everyone can decide how much they want on their kasha varnishkes, if any.*

JODIE'S QUINOA

This recipe was given to me by a patient who has brought all manner of wonderful foods to my office for me and my nurses over the years. They are always good and almost always plant-based, which this recipe can be if you use vegetable stock instead of chicken stock.

Yield: 4 servings

Ingredients:
- 1 cup diced onion
- 1 teaspoon minced garlic
- 2 tablespoons pine nuts (or other nuts)
- table salt, to taste
- ¼ teaspoon black pepper
- ¼ cup olive oil (preferably extra virgin)
- 1 cup dry quinoa
- 2 cups boiling chicken stock or vegetable stock, mixed with 2 tablespoons olive oil

Directions:

1. Throw the onion, garlic, and pine nuts, along with the salt and pepper, into a deep pot with the ½ cup of olive oil. Cook until the onion is transparent or slightly browned.
2. Place the quinoa in a fine mesh strainer and rinse under cold, running water until the water no longer foams. Add the quinoa to the onions and garlic and stir to distribute evenly.
3. Pour in the stock and oil mixture and cook for about 6–9 minutes until the liquid is absorbed.
4. Stir and fluff before serving.

SOFIA'S QUINOA WITH CHICKPEAS AND TOMATOES

This recipe is made by the delightful and helpful wife of a longtime patient of mine who has had to sharply change his eating habits due to some serious medical problems. As his doctor, I can attest to how much better he is now. Sofia went out of her way to make an Addictocarb-free meal for me when I was a dinner guest at their house one night, and I was just blown away by this dish. I asked her for the recipe, which she graciously provided.

Yield: 4 servings

Ingredients:

- 1 cup dry quinoa
- ⅛ teaspoon table salt, plus more to taste
- 1 ¾ cups water
- 1 cup canned chickpeas, drained
- 1 tomato, chopped
- 1 clove garlic, minced
- 3 tablespoons lime juice
- 4 teaspoons olive oil

- ½ teaspoon ground cumin
- black pepper, to taste
- ½ teaspoon chopped fresh parsley

1. Place the quinoa in a fine mesh strainer and rinse under cold, running water until the water no longer foams.
2. Put the quinoa, salt, and water in a saucepan and bring to a boil. Reduce heat to medium-low, cover, and let simmer until the quinoa is tender, about 20–25 minutes.
3. Once the quinoa is done, stir in the chickpeas, tomato, garlic, lime juice, and olive oil. Season with cumin, salt, and pepper. Sprinkle with parsley, then serve.

BEANS WITH PAN-FRIED CHICKEN OVER KASHA OR QUINOA

This is a fantastic Addictocarb Alternative to a rice meal, and you would be hard pressed to find a healthier or tastier meal anywhere. This recipe is interesting because it is basically bean soup without the soup, and it makes a beautiful and colorful presentation over a bed of kasha or quinoa. Your guests will gasp when they see it, and their eyes will light up when they taste it.

Yield: 4 servings

Ingredients:
- 1 package mixed dry beans (Goya makes a sixteen-bean mix available almost everywhere)
- 1 cup diced carrot
- 1 cup diced celery
- 1 cup diced onion
- 3 tablespoons chopped fresh parsley
- 1 tablespoon butter
- ½ cup olive oil, plus more for sautéing
- 6 cups chicken stock (preferably low sodium)

- 2 pounds thinly sliced chicken breasts
- 4 cups cooked kasha or quinoa, or more or less depending on your appetite (use the recipes in this section or just follow the recipe on the package)
- 1 tomato, sliced

1. Cover the dry beans with water and let soak overnight.
2. Sauté the carrot, celery, onion, and parsley in the butter and olive oil until soft, about 5 minutes.
3. Add the beans and vegetable mixture to the chicken stock. Heat to boiling, then turn down the heat and let simmer for 90 minutes.
4. Pour out most of the liquid from the soup, leaving just enough to keep the ingredients moist. Retain liquid for other uses (see tip below).
5. Sauté the chicken breasts in oil until they are cooked through.
6. For each serving, lay down a bed of about 1 cup of cooked kasha or quinoa, add a layer of the bean-vegetable mixture, and place a couple pieces of chicken breast on top of the whole thing. Garnish with half-slices of the tomato.

I would suggest drinking the leftover soup liquid as a broth, instead of having coffee or tea. It is very nutritious and will be delicious on a cold day or night.

CHAPTER 18

Other Recipes

OATMEAL

Oatmeal *can* be good for you, but the different types are confusing to the regular consumer like me. Like virtually every other food, the more it is processed the worse it is for you. For oatmeal, "processing" refers to breaking it into smaller and smaller pieces, steaming it, and even rolling it into flakes. Oat groats are the least processed, and instant oatmeal is the most processed. Steel-cut Irish oatmeal and Scottish oatmeal are the best compromise between processing and nutrition, and are the only kinds of oatmeal I recommend.

Yield: 4 servings

Ingredients
- 1 cup steel-cut oatmeal
- 1 sweetener, either mashed banana or apple (see recipes, page 130)

Directions:
1. Add the oatmeal to 4 cups of boiling water in a large pot.
2. Cook for about 30 minutes on low heat, mixing occasionally, until it has a creamy consistency.

3. Add one of the sweetener recipes using apples, pears, peaches, or bananas to taste. Serve hot.

ADDICTOCARB-FREE PANCAKES

I have fond memories of making my family Sunday morning breakfasts consisting of stacks of nutritious pancakes, which I took great pleasure in watching everyone gobble up. When I developed diabetes, I had to look for an alternative for these flour-laden treats. My nurse, Nicole, a food junkie herself, suggested banana pancakes. "How much flour do you put in?" I asked. "None," she said.

Intrigued I began to experiment. I added vanilla and cinnamon, a tasty as well as diabetes- and heart-friendly spice because it lowers blood sugar, triglycerides, and cholesterol.[1] I tried flaxseed, which helps reduce the risk of heart disease, cancer, stroke, and especially diabetes,[2] as well as gives substance to the mixture. I soon came to the realization that no matter what I put in these pancakes, they always come out tasting great.

Yield: 4 pancakes

Ingredients:
- 2 eggs (preferably organic, omega-3), beaten
- ¼ teaspoon ground cinnamon
- ¼ teaspoon vanilla extract
- 2 tablespoons flaxseed meal
- 2 small or 1 large ripe banana
- strawberries, peaches, or other fruit for topping (preferably organic)
- 2 tablespoons light pancake syrup (optional; no high fructose corn syrup) or apple sweetener (see page 130)

Directions:
1. In a bowl with the beaten eggs, add the cinnamon, vanilla extract, and flaxseed meal.

2. In a separate bowl, add the banana and mash it with an avocado or potato masher, or a fork. Make sure not to leave any lumps.

3. Add the egg mixture to the mashed bananas and mix well.

4. Lightly coat a skillet with cooking oil spray and set heat to medium-low (unlike regular pancakes, these can burn easily).

5. Ladle the mixture onto the skillet and watch it spread out just like a pancake.

6. Each pancake should only need to cook for a couple of minutes on each side. You will know when to turn it when you see the sides beginning to cook through, just like regular pancakes. Take great care in turning them because they are much lighter than flour-based pancakes.

7. Smother the pancakes with chopped fruit and, if you choose, add a tablespoon or two of light pancake syrup (I prefer Log Cabin® Lite, but lots of brands make similar kinds without high fructose corn syrup).

PUFFED BACON AND EGG NESTS

Chef James, a graduate of the famous Culinary Institute of America, works as a private chef. He is famous among my patients for his Breakfast Quinoa Oatmeal (page 162) and always comes up with recipes that not only adhere to the Addictocarb Diet lifestyle but are fascinating and often as much fun to read and prepare as they are to eat.

Yield: 4 nests

Ingredients:

- 4 eggs
- ½ teaspoon table salt, plus more to taste
- 2 tablespoons chopped chives
- ½ cup grated pecorino romano

- ½ cup cooked bacon, drained of grease
- black pepper, to taste

Directions:

1. Preheat the oven to 425°F.
2. Place parchment paper on a sheet pan and lightly coat with cooking spray.
3. Separate egg whites from the yolks. Reserve yolks in separate container or eggshells.
4. Place the egg whites and ½ teaspoon of salt in a stand mixer with a whisk attachment. Beat the egg whites, starting on low speed and working your way up to high speed, until stiff peaks form.
5. Gently fold in the cheese and chives.
6. Create four equal mounds of the egg white mixture on the lined baking sheet. Form the mounds so they look like nests, using the back of a spoon to make indentations in the centers.
7. Sprinkle the top of each nest with crumbled bacon.
8. Place the nests in the oven for 3–4 minutes until firm but not browned.
9. Remove baking sheet from the oven, gently add an egg yolk to the center of each nest, and season with salt and pepper.
10. Bake for 4 more minutes. Serve immediately.

BREAKFAST QUINOA OATMEAL

Here's another from recipe from Chef James. This recipe is perhaps the most famous and beloved recipe among my patients. I list it on my website (http://www.Addictocarb.com) and people just wax poetic about it. It is simple but elegant. While he uses sugar or Splenda, I personally prefer to use my apple or banana sweetener recipe (page 130).

Yield: 4 servings

Ingredients:

- 2 cups milk (preferably skim or almond)
- 1 cup dry quinoa, rinsed and drained
- 2 tablespoons sweetener (see page 130)
- ground cinnamon, to taste (usually ⅛–¼ teaspoon)
- ½–¾ cup fruit of your choice (preferably berries)

Directions:

1. Boil the milk.
2. Add quinoa and return to boil.
3. Reduce heat until almost all the liquid is absorbed, about 15 minutes.
4. Stir in sweetener and cinnamon to mix, and return to high heat for about 5 minutes.
5. Mix in fruit and serve warm.

LENTIL/PEA/BEAN SOUP WITH SOUR CREAM AND PICO DE GALLO

The thing about this lentil soup is that it does not really have to be lentil soup. The recipe works equally well as a pea soup or, my personal favorite, a sixteen-bean soup. The reason that I go out of my way to make this soup is that, unlike most lentil soups that you can buy, I put no potatoes in it, which makes it Addictocarb free. Also, if your diet is plant based, you can use vegetable stock instead of chicken. Nothing brilliant about this recipe, but it adheres to the tenets of the Addictocarb Diet and it tastes great.

Yield: 8 servings

Ingredients:

- 1 16-ounce package lentils, peas, black beans, or other dried beans (lentils do not have to be soaked overnight, but the other beans will cook faster if they are)

- 1 cup diced carrot
- 1 cup diced celery
- 1 cup diced onion
- 3 tablespoons chopped fresh parsley
- 1 tablespoon butter
- ½ cup olive oil
- 6 cups chicken or vegetable stock (preferably low sodium)
- 2 pounds chicken breasts, cooked (optional)
- 1 cup cooked kasha or quinoa
- ½ cup flaxseed meal (optional)
- 2 tablespoons sour cream per serving (optional)
- 2 tablespoons pico de gallo per serving (optional; page 164)

Directions:

1. Soak lentils, peas, or other beans overnight, then drain.
2. In a large pot, sauté the vegetables and parsley in the butter and olive oil until soft, about 5 minutes.
3. Add the beans and the chicken stock to the vegetable mixture, and bring to a boil. Then turn down the heat and let simmer for 90 minutes or until the beans are soft but still have some crunch to them.
4. After the soup is cooked, you can add a cup of cooked kasha or quinoa and a ½ cup of flaxseed meal.
5. Serve with sour cream and pico de gallo if desired.

- *You can make this soup into a really terrific dip by simply ladling about 1 cup into a food processor and blending until you have a smooth consistency. It tastes great with crudités.*
- *You can also serve it as a meal if you add chicken to it and serve it over a bed of kasha or quinoa.*

PICO DE GALLO

I use pico de gallo for just about everything, like bean soup (page 163), but also on top of guacamole (page 165), just plain on Wasa crackers or cucumber slices, and even straight up with a spoon out of the bowl. I rarely make it myself anymore because it has become so easy to get, freshly made, in virtually any supermarket. But here it is anyway.

Yield: 2 cups

Ingredients:
- 2 cups diced tomatoes
- ¼ cup diced onion (Vidalia™ or red preferably)
- about 1 tablespoon diced jalapenos or 1/8 teaspoon Tabasco®, depending on how hot you like things
- 1 tablespoon minced garlic
- 1 tablespoon lime or lemon juice, fresh or bottled
- 3–5 tablespoons cilantro, to taste
- table salt and black pepper, to taste

Directions:
1. Throw everything into a bowl and toss.

GUACAMOLE

At the risk of sounding full of myself, I must say that I am famous for my guacamole. Everyone we know requests it when they come over, including my kids, who like to order it up before they visit. It's always a big hit at backyard parties and just as good in a pinch for dinner or an after-school/after-work snack.

In the old days I made tacos and burritos for the kids with it, but these days I just eat it plain or with Wasa Crisp'n Light Crackerbreads, and even on cucumber slices, and it's just as good. This guacamole is packed with antioxidants, is good for diabetes, and is one of the true taste sensations on the planet.

Yield: 4 servings

Ingredients:

- 2 avocados
- ½ onion, finely diced
- 3 tablespoons finely chopped fresh cilantro
- juice of ½ lime or ¼ lemon, or 1 teaspoon lemon juice concentrate
- ¼ teaspoon Tabasco sauce or other hot sauce
- 1 small tomato, diced small
- Wasa Crisp'n Light Crackerbreads

Directions:

1. Cut the avocados in half and remove the pits. Scoop out the flesh and put it in a bowl.
2. Mash the avocado with an avocado or potato masher or a fork.
3. Mix in the onion and cilantro.
4. Add the lime or lemon juice and Tabasco and mix.
5. Add the diced tomato and mix carefully so you don't destroy the integrity of the tomato.
6. Serve immediately with the crackerbreads.

TOMATOES, MOZZARELLA, AVOCADO, AND ONION WITH OLIVE OIL

This recipe is pretty much a staple for me, as it is for many people. It is easy to put together and never disappoints. The biggest and most difficult decision for me every time I make it is whether to use cilantro or basil. Either one is great, and there's not an Addictocarb in sight.

Yield: 4 side dish servings; 1 meal serving

Ingredients:

- 1 tomato, sliced
- 1 large fresh mozzarella ball, thinly sliced

- 1 avocado, sliced
- 1 onion (I prefer Vidalia™), *very* thinly sliced
- ¼ cup coarsely chopped fresh cilantro or basil
- extra-virgin olive oil to drizzle
- kosher salt, to taste
- black pepper, to taste

Directions:

1. Place a slice of tomato on a plate and add slices of mozzarella, avocado, and onion on top, alternating and taking care to drizzle olive oil and place cilantro or basil between each layer. Top it off with salt and pepper to taste.

IRISH KALE BURGER

This transcendent recipe, given to me by Jeannette Gamble, a patient and a food blogger with a brogue to match her burger, truly embodies the essence of the Addictocarb Diet. The squash bun is beyond brilliant. This recipe may be just as much fun to read as to cook, but it is definitely fun to eat. Visit her blog at www.jgamble-food.com, where she also has great pictures. In her own words:

For those of you who have visited Ireland, what is most striking is the countryside and vast areas of green landscapes. There are layers of color that all blend to make a perfect picture, and they are the inspiration for how I approach plating my dishes. Two years ago I suffered from an extreme knee injury, which took a great deal of time to recover from. My grandmother, who is an amazing cook, took it upon herself to look after me during this time. She knew my love for a simple burger, but in an effort to nurse me back to health she removed all carbohydrates from the dish and made a beautiful kale burger with a bun that was made out of squash. All the ingredients were sourced from the fields in County Fermanagh and created with patience and love. The Irish Kale Burger is a celebration of my Irish heritage and my grandmother.

Yield: 4 large or 6 medium burgers

Ingredients:
- 1 small winter squash
- 1 pound grass-fed ground beef
- 1 small red onion, diced small
- 2 cloves garlic, finely minced
- 2 bunches kale, finely chopped
- 5 tablespoons fiery salsa, plus more for topping
- 1 egg yolk (large egg)
- ½ teaspoon chili or red pepper flakes
- sea salt, to taste
- freshly ground black pepper, to taste
- 1–2 tablespoons pure Irish butter (preferably Kerrygold)
- 1 small white onion, roughly diced
- 1 avocado, thinly sliced

Directions:
1. Preheat the oven to 400°F.
2. Remove the skin of the squash and scoop out the seeds. Dice into ½-inch pieces. Place in a roasting dish and roast for approximately 20 minutes until soft.
3. In a large mixing bowl, combine the ground beef, red onion, garlic, kale, salsa, egg yolk, chili or red pepper flakes, and salt and pepper and mix thoroughly. Make sure all the ingredients are chopped evenly and well mixed through, or the burger will not cook properly.
4. Divide the meat mixture into 4 portions (or 6 for smaller burgers). Using your hands, gently form each portion into a ball shape, making sure not to overwork the meat.

5. In a frying pan over medium-high heat, fry the white onion in the butter until caramelized, achieving a nice browning effect. Then set aside.

6. Heat the frying pan on high heat for 1 minute, then reduce it to medium-high and add the burgers to the pan. Do not touch the burgers once you have them in the frying pan. Cook them until golden brown and slightly charred on the first side, about 3 minutes, then flip them. Cook until golden brown and slightly charred on the second side, about 3 minutes, for medium rare or until desired doneness.

7. Take the squash out of the oven and mash with an avocado or potato masher or a fork. Then use your hands or a patty maker (see tip below) to shape the squash into the "buns" for your burgers.

8. To assemble the burgers, put one of the squash buns in the middle of a plate. Top with a burger and align them perfectly. Layer the avocado slices on top of the burger, add some caramelized onion, and top with salsa. You can either leave the burger open or add an additional layer of squash on top.

Someone gave me a fancy burger maker that makes all my burgers the perfect shape and width, but you can just use your hands. You can also search on Amazon for a burger maker or patty press. They range from $8 to $20.

NICOLE'S DAD'S ADDICTOCARB-FREE EGGPLANT PARMESAN

Nicole, my nurse, has been transformed from chubby to svelte on her diet, helped along by her father, a Romanian chef. He has gone out of his way to come up with recipes that fit the Addictocarb Diet way of life. I always look forward to the days she brings in her lunch and warms it up in the microwave. The aroma sends me to another place.

Yield: 4 servings

Ingredients:
- 1 large eggplant, sliced lengthwise about ¼-inch thick
- table salt, for removing liquid from eggplant and to taste
- black pepper, to taste
- ¼ cup olive oil (preferably virgin), plus more to drizzle
- 1 cup chopped onion
- 2 cloves garlic, minced
- 4–5 leaves fresh basil, coarsely chopped
- 1 28-ounce can Italian tomatoes (preferably San Marzano)
- 2 cups grated parmesan cheese (preferably reggiano), divided
- ½ pound mozzarella cheese, thinly sliced or grated

Directions:
1. Preheat the oven to 375°F and coat a baking sheet with nonstick spray.
2. Salt the eggplant slices generously, then let them sit for about half an hour so the bitter liquid is drawn out. Rinse the salt off and pat dry with paper towels.
3. Place the eggplant slices on the baking sheet, add fresh ground black pepper to taste, and drizzle with a bit of olive oil. Bake for 10–15 minutes until slightly browned. Then turn over and bake for another 10 minutes.
4. While the eggplant is baking, add the ¼ cup of olive oil to a medium saucepan and heat on medium for 1 minute.
5. Add the onion and cook for 2–3 minutes until the onion is translucent.
6. Add the garlic and basil and cook for 1 minute.
7. Add the tomatoes along with their juice. Lower the heat, add salt to taste, and let simmer for about half an hour. Then let the sauce cool.
8. To assemble the eggplant parmesan, layer bottom of a glass baking dish (9″ × 5″, 8″ × 8″, or 9″ × 13″) with the tomato sauce, just enough to coat.

9. Add a layer of eggplant slices on top of the sauce and dust the eggplant with parmesan cheese.
10. Repeat with a layer of sauce, followed by eggplant and parmesan. Keep doing this until you run out of eggplant or space in the dish. Top with fresh mozzarella cheese.
11. Turn the oven down to 250°F and bake for about 25 minutes. The eggplant and sauce are already cooked, so this is mostly to seal the flavors together and melt the cheeses. If you like a crispy top, put it on broil for the last 2 minutes or so, but watch it closely! You don't want to over-broil it and have a charred top.

THE OTHER ELLEN'S ROASTED HERB SALMON

For a couple of decades, every time my patient Ellen called my office or spoke to me on the phone, she pointed out that "it is the other Ellen" to make sure I did not confuse her with my wife, who is also named Ellen. I never have, but it has become a standing joke at my office. Also, over the years we have talked on and on about our struggles with our weight. Now we are both skinny, and "the other Ellen" has clearly distinguished herself with this recipe. It is easy, delicious, and Addictocarb free.

Yield: 4 servings

Ingredients:
- 2 pounds skinless salmon fillet
- table salt and black pepper, to taste
- ¼ cup olive oil
- 2 tablespoons lemon juice
- ½ cup minced fresh scallions
- ½ cup minced fresh dill
- ½ cup minced fresh parsley
- ¼ cup dry white wine

Directions:

1. Preheat oven to 425°F.
2. Season salmon generously with salt and pepper and place in a ceramic, glass, or stainless steel roasting dish.
3. Whisk olive oil and lemon juice together, then coat the salmon fillet with the mixture.
4. Allow salmon to rest at room temperature for 15–20 minutes.
5. In a bowl, combine the minced scallions, dill, and parsley. Gently spread the mixture evenly over the salmon. Then pour white wine around and over salmon.
6. Roast the salmon for 10–12 minutes. The center should be slightly pinker than the rest of the filet.
7. Remove from oven and cover with aluminum foil for 10 minutes before serving.

LUCIE'S SALMON

This recipe was given to me by a friend who has been astounding my family with her cooking prowess for years. She has a habit of always living near the water and so she has the opportunity and the knack for cooking interesting fresh fish recipes. It is hard to tell if her French accent improves the dish, but one thing is for sure: This dish is great even without it. She has been supportive of the Addictocarb-free lifestyle from the very beginning, and this dish fits it perfectly.

Yield: 4 servings

Ingredients:

- 1 ½ pounds salmon fillets
- ¼ teaspoon kosher salt
- ⅛ teaspoon black pepper
- 3 tablespoons grated fresh ginger
- 4 scallions, cut into 6-inch juliennes

- 2 tablespoons olive oil
- 2 tablespoons Kikkoman® lime-flavored ponzu sauce
- cooked quinoa

Directions:

1. Preheat oven to 375°F and line a cookie sheet with an 18-inch-long sheet of parchment paper.
2. Wash the salmon fillets, pat them dry, and arrange them skin side down on the lined baking sheet.
3. Season the fillets with salt and pepper, and then spread the grated ginger on top.
4. Arrange the julienned scallions on top of the fish and drizzle it with olive oil and ponzu sauce.
5. Fold the parchment paper, starting with the long sides, then fold the ends until sealed, and press firmly.
6. Bake for 30 minutes. Then carefully open the parchment paper and serve the fillets with quinoa.

JODIE'S SALMON

Jodie, as I have mentioned before, is just chock full of great recipes that she has been bringing in for me and my nurses for years. This is just one more.

Yield: 2 servings

Ingredients:

- 1 pound fresh salmon, rinsed and dried

Marinade

- 1 tablespoon toasted or plain sesame oil
- 2 tablespoons olive oil
- 1 tablespoon low-sodium soy sauce
- 1 teaspoon apple cider vinegar
- 2 teaspoons rice wine vinegar

- ¼ teaspoon black pepper
- ⅛ teaspoon crushed red pepper flakes
- ¾ teaspoon five spice powder
- 1–2 cloves garlic, crushed or minced
- 1 teaspoon grated fresh ginger

Directions:

1. In a bowl, whisk the sesame oil, olive oil, soy sauce, vinegars, black and red pepper, five spice powder, garlic, and ginger until blended, and pour into a resealable plastic bag.
2. Place salmon in the bag and swish it around to coat the fish on all sides.
3. Marinate in the fridge for 2 hours.
4. Preheat the oven to 450°F.
5. Place the salmon, skin side down, in a nonstick pan and bake until cooked through, about 12 minutes. It should go from its original bright color to a duller pinkish color. Insert the tip of a knife into the thickest part of the fish and then touch it to your lip. If it is hot, then the fish is done; if not, cook it some more. When it is done, the fish should be flaky, which means that if you put a fork between the grooves in the fish, it should come apart easily.

ROBIN'S WORLD'S BEST MEATLOAF

Making house calls over the years has treated me to all types of great foods that patients often have waiting for me, and I love it. At one time, it was freshly baked cakes, breads, and truffles that delighted me, but now I have other priorities.

One day while making a house call to see an elderly patient that my nurse and I refer to as Oma (which is apparently Dutch for "grandma"), I was suddenly overtaken by the most unbelievable aroma. On my way out of the house I could not help myself and poked my nose in the kitchen where Oma's daughter-in-law, Robin, was in the midst of making the most unusual meatloaf I had ever seen. After a quick assessment to make sure there were no Addictocarbs in sight, I asked for the recipe. She said, "I will do more than that," and she did. The next day she dropped off a gigantic piece of meatloaf at my office along with the recipe. I can only say that when she calls it "the world's best meatloaf," she is not kidding around.

Yield: 6 servings

Ingredients:
- 1 ½ pounds carrots, thinly sliced
- 1 onion, diced
- 3 tablespoons olive oil
- 1 teaspoon ground cinnamon
- 1 teaspoon ground nutmeg
- ½ teaspoon ginger powder
- 1 pound ground beef or turkey
- 2 eggs, beaten
- ¼ cup milk (skim, almond, or soy)
- 1 teaspoon dried thyme
- ½ cup chopped fresh cilantro or parsley
- organic ketchup (no high fructose corn syrup)

Directions:
1. Preheat the oven to 350°F.
2. Cook the sliced carrots until soft, about 7–9 minutes in a pot of boiling water or microwaved in 2 tablespoons of water for about 6–9 minutes. You can also steam them for about 10 minutes.
3. Sauté the onion in olive oil until soft, about 5 minutes.

4. In a bowl, place the cooked carrots and onions, and add the cinnamon, nutmeg, and ginger. Mash everything with an avocado or potato masher until well mixed.

5. In a separate bowl, mix the ground meat with the beaten eggs, milk, thyme, and cilantro or parsley.

6. Cover a 15-inch piece of wax paper with cooking spray and lay out the meat mixture in a flat rectangle that will be easy to roll.

7. Place the carrot and onion mixture on top of the meat in an even layer, and then roll it by lifting the wax paper from the back, just like a jelly roll.

8. After the meatloaf is all rolled up, place it on a greased cookie sheet. Brush the entire surface with ketchup and bake it in the oven for 50 minutes.

FRUIT SALAD

It doesn't get any better than this. This recipe is extremely healthy, tasty, high carb, high calorie, and, best of all, Addictocarb free, so you'll have no cravings afterward.

Yield: 4 servings

Ingredients:
- raspberries, amount as desired
- strawberries, amount as desired
- blueberries, amount as desired
- prunes, diced, amount as desired
- ½ apple, cored and cut into 1-inch pieces
- ½ pear, cut into 1-inch pieces
- ½ cup Stonyfield® or Greek yogurt (low fat or 0%)

Directions:
1. Mix the fruit in a large bowl and add in the yogurt. Mix gently so you don't bruise the fruit. Peel the apples and pears unless they are organic.

APPLESAUCE

··

This is a healthy, Addictocarb-free, antioxidant-laden, non-fattening food, and it is great for diabetics. I originally came up with this recipe for my children, since I did not like feeding them store-bought applesauce. I used to make extra and put the leftover in ice cube trays so that I could warm up a cube anytime my kids were hungry.

The problem with most commercial applesauces is that many contain added sugar. The apples you buy, like pears and peaches, should really be organic; at the very least, wash them carefully and peel them before eating or making them into sauce.

Applesauce is one of the easiest things to make, and if you make it this way, you can even serve it to babies. This recipe is perhaps the easiest in the book.

Yield: 4 servings

Ingredients:

- 3 apples, peeled, cored, and cut into 2-inch pieces
- ¼ teaspoon ground cinnamon (optional)
- 5–10 berries (optional)

Directions:

1. Place the apple pieces, cinnamon if using, and berries if using, into a food processor and pulse them on high for about 60 seconds or until the apples have the consistency of applesauce. Adults may like it chunky, but if you are giving it to babies it has to be really smooth.

Applesauce tastes great on latkes, sweet potato pancakes, or just about any sweet potato food. It is also a fine non-Addictocarb snack on its own, and of course it is great for babies. I tell new parents to put the applesauce in an ice cube tray and, when it is frozen, store the cubes in a plastic bag so you can take them out whenever you need them. Just nuke them in the microwave for a few seconds or allow them to defrost naturally.

CHOCOLATE-POWDERED STRAWBERRIES

This Addictocarb-free recipe is beyond simple, tastes great, and is a welcome snack or dessert anytime—after dinner or at halftime during the Super Bowl. It is a great idea for someone who absolutely, positively has to have something sweet.

Yield: 10 strawberries

Ingredients:
- 10 large strawberries
- 1 scoop Slimfast or other brand chocolate powder discussed earlier (page 51)

Directions:
1. Slice the strawberries about ¼-inch thick and lay them out on a plate.
2. Sprinkle the chocolate powder over the strawberries and serve.

RANI'S CILANTRO POPCORN

Rani is not a patient. She is my wife's friend, who over recent years had gained a lot of weight. Since my wife and I are constantly marveling at the success of the Addictocarb Diet, she decided to subscribe to some of its tenets. All I can say is that she has lost more than twenty-five pounds and looks like a different person, which I would say qualifies her as an Addictocarb Diet lifestyle expert.

She once asked me if popcorn was okay on the diet. I said yes, and this is her personalized take on it. It fits the Addictocarb Diet quite well: high carb, high fiber, whole grain, low glycemic index, and, most importantly, nonaddictive. She makes it using an air popper but you can also just pop it in a paper bag in the microwave.

Stay away from the popular store-bought microwave popcorns. They often have all sorts of stuff in them that is not good for you.

Yield: 3 cups

Ingredients:

- ¼ cup organic popcorn kernels
- 1 tablespoon parmesan cheese
- kosher salt, to taste
- ¼ teaspoon lemon-pepper spice
- 10 large leaves basil or one handful cilantro, minced

Directions:

1. If using an air popper, add the kernels and pop. If using a microwave, place the kernels in a paper bag and fold the top over a few times. Place the bag upright into the microwave and heat on high for about 2 minutes or until you hear the corn stop popping.
2. Put the popcorn in a large bowl and sprinkle the remaining ingredients over it. Give the bowl a few shakes and serve.

AARON'S OUTDOOR BARBECUE-GRILLED PINEAPPLE AND PEACHES

My son Aaron, who is skinny, discovered grilled fruit at college. I tasted it and liked it, and so here it is. While he uses peaches and pineapple, I believe you could grill just about any fruit and it would be terrific and Addictocarb free.

Yield: 4–6 servings

Ingredients:

- 1 fresh pineapple, cored
- 3 fresh peaches

Directions:

1. Slice the pineapple and peaches.
2. Throw them on the grill and cook for 2 minutes on each side.

CHAPTER 19

Sample Menus

I have mixed feelings about providing sample menus. On one hand, I think it can be helpful to see what it is possible to eat from the standpoint of the Addictocarb Diet. On the other hand, I firmly believe, as I have said in the book, that you should only eat when you are hungry. And if you are only going to eat when you are hungry, that does away with the idea of breakfast, lunch, and dinner. You *can* miss meals and it is no problem. Also, how much you eat should be based on how hungry you are. I often will eat nothing but an entire bag of sweet potato fries and a glass of the Shake for dinner. Why not? It is extremely healthy, tasty, filling, good for my diabetes, and easy to prepare. I do not feel that I need to observe the convention of sitting down to three meals a day and serving an appetizer, a main course, and a dessert.

It has been shown repeatedly that one big difference between fat people and skinny people is that skinny people eat when they are hungry and fat people eat on cues: "It is dinner time, so let's eat," or, "It is a birthday party, so let's gorge ourselves." The reality is, you should eat whenever you want, and as much as you want, as long as you take care to eat the right things.

So, with all that being said, here is a week's worth of sample menus. Use them as you will.

Day 1

Breakfast

nonfat Greek yogurt (6 ounces), walnuts, berries
(raspberries, blueberries, and strawberries), with a
Shake

Lunch

Basil, Ham, and Cheese Sandwich (page 131) and
strawberries (see "Berries and Burgers"
on page 55)

Dinner

Plain and Easy Tomato Sauce (page 149) with
Dreamfields pasta and all the vegetables you want
(broccoli, cauliflower, spinach, carrots,
sweet potatoes, etc.)
Any size salad you want with oil and vinegar salad
dressing, lettuce, tomatoes, avocado, onions,
and carrots

Snack

fruits (apples, pears, peaches, grapes, strawberries,
blueberries, etc.)
Special Snack of the Day: handful of peanuts

Day 2

Breakfast

peanuts, almonds, and prunes with a Shake

Lunch

Guacamole (page 165) with 3 Wasa Crisp'n Light 7
Grain Crackerbreads

Dinner

Nicole's Dad's Addictocarb-Free Eggplant Parmesan
(page 169) and all the vegetables you want (broccoli,
cauliflower, spinach, carrots, sweet potatoes, etc.)
Any size salad you want with oil and vinegar salad
dressing, lettuce, tomatoes, avocado, onions, and
carrots

Snack

fruits (apples, pears, peaches, grapes, strawberries,
blueberries, etc.)
Special Snack of the Day: 1–2 cups popcorn

Day 3

Breakfast

Peanut Butter and Raspberries Sandwich (page 134)
with a Shake

Lunch

Celery Dill Tuna Sandwich (page 133)

Dinner

Jodie's Quinoa (page 155) with Pan-Fried Chicken
(page 157) and all the vegetables you want (broccoli,
cauliflower, spinach, carrots, sweet potatoes, etc.)
Any size salad you want with oil and vinegar salad
dressing, lettuce, tomatoes, avocado, onions,
and carrots

Snack

fruits (apples, pears, peaches, grapes, strawberries,
blueberries, etc.)
Special snack of the day: 2 one-inch squares dark
chocolate (72 percent cacao)

$\mathcal{D}ay\ 4$

Breakfast

3 Wasa Crisp'n Light 7 Grain Crackerbreads
with a Shake

Lunch

My Favorite Roast Beef Sandwich (page 132) with
berries (see "Berries and Burgers" on page 55)

Dinner

Irish Kale Burger (page 167) with berries
Wendy's Mashed Unpotato (page 142) and all the
vegetables you want (broccoli, cauliflower, spinach,
carrots, sweet potatoes, etc.)
Any size salad you want with oil and vinegar salad
dressing, lettuce, tomatoes, avocado, onions,
and carrots

Snack

fruits (apples, pears, peaches, grapes, strawberries,
blueberries, etc.)
Special Snack of the Day: cherry tomatoes

Day 5

Breakfast

Breakfast Quinoa Oatmeal (page 162)

Lunch

Garlic Fried Spaghetti (page 147)

Dinner

Cauliflower Pizza (page 137) and all the vegetables
you want (broccoli, cauliflower, spinach, carrots,
sweet potatoes, etc.)
Any size salad you want with oil and vinegar salad
dressing, lettuce, tomatoes, avocado, onions,
and carrots

Snack

fruits (apples, pears, peaches, grapes, strawberries,
blueberries, etc.)
Special Snack of the Day: 5 large luscious dark
chocolate–covered almonds

Day 6

Breakfast

Addictocarb-Free Pancakes (page 160)

Lunch

Garlic Fried Spaghetti (page 147)

Dinner

My Personal Bolognese Sauce (page 151) with
Dreamfields pasta or eaten as a chili with berries
(see "Berries and Burgers" on page 55) and all the
vegetables you want (broccoli, cauliflower, spinach,
carrots, sweet potatoes, etc.)
Any size salad you want with oil and vinegar
salad dressing, lettuce, tomatoes, avocado, onions,
and carrots

Snack

fruits (apples, pears, peaches, grapes, strawberries,
blueberries, etc.)
Special Snack of the Day: handful of walnuts

Day 7

Breakfast

bacon and eggs with strawberries (see "Berries
and Burgers" on page 55)

Lunch

Basil, Ham, and Cheese Sandwich (page 131)
and a Shake

Dinner

Fruit Salad (page 176) with 3 Wasa Crisp'n Light
7 Grain Crackerbreads and all the vegetables you
want (broccoli, cauliflower, spinach, carrots,
sweet potatoes, etc.)
Any size salad you want with oil and vinegar salad
dressing, lettuce, tomatoes, avocado, onions,
and carrots

Snack

fruits (apples, pears, peaches, grapes, strawberries,
blueberries, etc.)
Special Snack of the Day: Chocolate-Powdered
Strawberries (page 178)

APPENDICES

APPENDIX A

Your Frequently
Asked Questions

've prepared this appendix based on the most common questions from hundreds of my patients who have tried the Addictocarb Diet. As this book receives wide circulation, I expect new questions will arise, so I am incorporating these and all future frequently asked questions into a page on my website (http://www.Addictocarb.com/questions.html). Please visit the site and feel free to add your own questions.

GENERAL QUESTIONS

I need to lose weight quickly in order to motivate myself or by a certain date. What should I do?
I get asked this question constantly. Losing a couple of pounds a week is fine; two pounds a week will total 104 pounds in the first year and even one pound per week works out to 52 pounds a year. Yet, as a doctor, I realize that I must treat patients within the restrictions that they place on me. I can tell patients that losing weight slowly is good and healthy, but if they do not accept that, then I must work within their parameters.

If you must lose weight faster to motivate yourself, or for other timely reasons like an upcoming wedding, class reunion, or audition, then I do have a pat solution that I give my patients. Let me illustrate the point by telling you a story about a patient that I have been taking care of for a very long time who put this question to me. Let me also mention that she lost more than twenty pounds and three dress sizes on the Addictocarb Diet.

A friend came to visit us from South Carolina; she asked my wife if she could see a certain Broadway show. The patient I just mentioned was, coincidentally, the associate director of the show, so I called and asked her if she could arrange house seats for us and perhaps give our friend a backstage tour. She was extremely gracious, and after the show we went backstage to meet the cast. Our friend just thought it was the greatest thing ever. My wife was thrilled. Everyone was happy—except me.

When I saw my patient backstage, I was astonished to see how much weight she had gained. I was terribly upset because this was a woman that I had watched sing and dance as a star on Broadway just a few years previously. After she took my wife and her friend on the tour, and as we were planning to leave, I pulled her aside and suggested to her that she had to do something. She nodded and she said she would call me, which she did.

She recounted for me her arduous journey from ingénue to choreographer, and now to associate director of a major Broadway show, while at the same time getting married and having children. She had gained about forty pounds. While she had never had a serious weight issue, keeping her weight down had always been a matter of some contention due to the intense demands of the entertainment industry. Forty pounds was a problem, and she knew it. She was having trouble keeping up with her children, and while she was considering opening a touring company in Chicago, she wondered if she had the energy to do it, even though it would be a financial boon and a professional accomplishment. She also said something that cut me to the quick: When she looked at her two daughters, she was overwhelmed with emotion, worrying that she would not be able to dance at their weddings. She wanted to be there for them. It reminded me of my father's absence at my wedding due to his premature death.

I suggested that if she really wanted to lose weight quickly, she should substitute water for milk in her Shakes and leave out the banana. She thought that was a great idea, pointing out to me that she had problems with milk. After speaking with me and making the switch in her Shake, she lost eight pounds in the first week, and she was committed. At that point I told her she could switch to almond or soy milk and restore the banana, but she was fine with exactly what she had been doing, so why mess with success?

She has always been good about keeping me updated on how she is doing on the diet. As I was writing this book, she had lost more than twenty pounds and was fully committed to her forty-pound weight loss goal. However, the important thing is that she feels she has conquered her addiction and does not feel compelled to eat the way she had in recent years. She has fallen off the wagon a few times, but with the help of the Shakes and staying off Addictocarbs, she has been able to get back on track. Not only is she determined to lose another twenty pounds, but now, having conquered her addiction, she does not feel it is going to be hard. That is the beauty of conquering your food addiction.

So, finally, what is my pat answer to a patient's plea to lose weight faster? While I do not necessarily recommend it, it is to substitute water or almond milk for cow's milk in the Shake, leave out the banana, and even leave out the flavoring powder.

Is it true I do not have to worry about quantities of food?
Yes, it is entirely true. It is liberating to simply know exactly which foods you cannot eat and to be able to eat everything

else in whatever quantities you want. Remember that the list of Addictocarbs is small compared to the number of available foods.

What is the success rate of the diet?

I have counseled close to a thousand people on the Addictocarb Diet over the past decade. The success rate has been astounding. I would say that about 80 percent of the people that go on my diet lose weight and very many of them keep much of it off. Over time, virtually everyone who goes on the diet develops a basic understanding of how to eat. When I put someone on the diet, I make sure to tell them to call me on a regular basis to keep me up to date on their progress. You can do this for yourself by simply filling out *The Addictocarb Diet* Progress Tool in Appendix D (page 213).

When people have a relapse, I simply encourage them to go right back on the diet. I go out of my way to explain that this is more of a lifestyle change than just a diet. This book contains everything I tell my patients, and I intend for it to be used as a substitute for me. When you have questions, it is likely that my patients have had the same questions, and you can consult the book to find the answers. You can also reread sections of the book to remind you of the tenets of the diet. The website is also helpful on this point (http://www.Addictocarb.com), and I am always happy to read people's stories there.

Do calories and carbs matter?

In terms of the Addictocarb Diet, no, they do not. Why? Because the basis of this diet is that by reducing your cravings you will eat less. It works. I know that. My patients know that. That being said, however, the reality is that total calories and carbs count. However, if you follow everything established in *The Addictocarb Diet* you will simply end up eating fewer calories because you will have fewer cravings; and since you are eliminating Addictocarbs, you are cutting out most of the carbohydrates you previously consumed. Over the years I have watched countless people lose weight and keep it off without watching calories and carbs just by staying on the Addictocarb Diet.

What about the glycemic index?

The glycemic index, which measures how much of and how quickly food is broken down into sugar and absorbed into the bloodstream, is a good way to gauge whether a food is fattening or bad for you. On the other hand, if you are following a low-glycemic diet, that would rule out eating the amount of fruit recommended for the Addictocarb Diet. If you stick to the Addictocarb Diet, you will not have to worry about the glycemic index. It is too difficult to have to deal with all those numbers. The Addictocarb Diet is easier and will cut out most of the high-glycemic foods anyway.

How quickly will I lose weight?

The most important thing to understand is to not live and die by the scale. Let's say you lose four pounds per month, which works out to only about a pound a week, which would be about fifty pounds in a year. By anybody's account, that is a lot of weight to lose. But even if you lost two pounds per month—only a half of a pound per week—that would still be about twenty-five pounds per year.

So how much weight do you really want to lose? You will be able to lose as much as you want, but that will require some decision making on your part. Do you want to give up all Addictocarbs, or do you want to give up some of them? Maybe just giving up one of them is enough for you. Remember, the point of this diet is not exclusively to lose weight but also to keep the weight off. So all that being said, I would say that losing about four pounds per month is optimal. Some people lose more and are still not satisfied, and some people lose less and are thrilled.

How often should I weigh myself?

There are studies, such as one in the *Annals of Behavioral Medicine* titled "Self-Weighing in Weight Gain Prevention and Weight Loss Trials," that have shown that people who weigh themselves daily lose more weight on diets.[1] I am personally opposed to this. As I have stated repeatedly in this book, if you want to lose a lot of weight quickly, just go on the Atkins Diet or almost any fad diet. You will lose weight, with many of them even quite quickly. Repeatedly weighing yourself may actually help with those diets, *but* the point of the Addictocarb Diet is not to lose weight quickly only to put it back on again just as quickly. It is to conquer your food addiction so that you can lose weight *and* stay slim for the rest of your life.

So how often do I feel you should weigh yourself? I would say that once a month would be plenty, but everyone is different. You will know if you are losing weight by how your clothes fit and if you are just generally feeling better. If you are getting thinner, other people will notice and mention it to you. You do not need to live and die by the scale.

LIFESTYLE

What can I eat at a Mexican restaurant?

I got a call from a patient one day who was doing great on the diet and had lost twelve or fifteen pounds already. She was in a Mexican restaurant and was wondering if she could have chips with salsa. I texted her back, "Absolutely no chips." Chips are Addictocarbs. Then before I sent her some suggestions, I thought back to the Super Bowl of that year, where the NFL threw a lavish Mexican-themed food party, which I was lucky enough to attend, and I did very well Addictocarb Diet–wise. I simply suggested to her what had already worked for me.

Almost everything at a Mexican restaurant is wrapped or served with Addictocarb-laden chips, tortillas, or wraps.

However, most of these dishes may be easily modified so you can stay on the diet. For instance, fajitas can be eaten without the tortillas. You can skip the rice as well. Beans are healthy. Queso flameado, which is just beef and cheese, is great as long as it is eaten without the chips. All in all, you can have an excellent and satisfying Mexican meal without the Addictocarbs.

I work in an office all week for ten hours a day. What do I do during Step 1 if I can't make Shakes?

My patients have come up with all sorts of ways to deal with this. I am always impressed by the number of patients that walk into my office carrying all manner of portable containers. I am actually fascinated by the technology that I had not previously even considered. One patient who had to be at work every day came up with another ingenious method. She made a fruit-slushy concentrate by whipping up her fruits in a blender and then putting them in a thermos. Once at work she would expand her fruit slush by adding either water or milk. This worked extremely well for her, and I have recommended to other patients who report success.

Other patients have mentioned that they just bring one of those little blenders, like the Bullet, to work.

Thermos® makes a slew of drink bottles, and the most useful sizes for the diet are 34 ounces (1 liter), 68 ounces (2 liters), and my personal favorite, 48 ounces (1.4 liters), because it perfectly fits the Shake from my blender.

I'm on the road 60 percent of the time for business. How do I manage this diet?

If we are talking about fast food, I deal with that in chapter ten, "Fast Food the Addictocarb Diet Way" (page 97). In terms of going out for dinner, see my strategies in chapter eight, "Getting Back 'On the Wagon'" (page 83).

I'm a stay-at-home parent with three kids and a hungry spouse. How do I stick to a diet like this when I prepare meals and I'm totally outnumbered?

No problem. I can tell you from my own family and the families of many of my patients that they will not know the difference when you substitute Dreamfields pasta for any other pasta. Also, you may find that the family enjoys things like kasha or quinoa. Especially in the case of French fries, you will find that sweet potato fries are perfectly acceptable to the rest of the family. One point of this diet is that it is healthy for you; it will also be healthy for your children and spouse. So, in short, I think you will find that this is easier than you think.

If I skip breakfast, won't I be starving later and then overeat?

NO! See my full explanation of this in chapter four, "Two Rules to Help You Lose Weight and Keep It Off" (page 37).

SPECIFIC FOOD QUESTIONS

What if I am not sure if I can eat a certain food?

In a pinch, assuming you cannot find someone to ask or cannot access my website, you can always turn to the total calorie count, carb count, glycemic index, and total sugars. This is not ideal because there are certain things these measures would restrict, like fruit, and certain things they would allow, like bread. For instance, if you are not sure which yogurt you can eat, you can check the calorie count, carb content, and sugar content of all the yogurts on the store shelf. You will be surprised at how many different brands there are and how different the calories and carbs and glycemic index are. There are also convenient books and great mobile apps for looking up these things. For instance, CalorieKing® has an app for your phone that is easy to use.

What if I need something sweet?

This is a common question among people on most diets, and when they ask me this question, I know it is because of their experience with other diets. With other diets that ask you to limit certain foods, the addiction center of the brain is still stimulated. With this diet, by totally abstaining from the various Addictocarbs, cravings will not be such an issue. I remember one patient said to me after just three days, "I am shocked by how little I feel compelled to eat Addictocarbs." This same sentiment has been expressed to me more times that I can count. Nevertheless, because this is a common question, here is my answer: If the vast variety of fruits is not enough, try Greek yogurt like Chobani® or FAGE® or a couple of squares of 72 percent dark chocolate. You can also make hot chocolate using just Slimfast or the protein powder of your choice, and you will be pleased by how good it tastes and how little it stimulates your addiction center. Another thing I often recommend is my Chocolate-Powdered Strawberries recipe (page 178). Last, in the recipes section I have recipes for "sweeteners," which are basically blended whole fruit.

What about peanuts?

Peanuts are fattening, but if you stick to eating around nine peanuts at a crack it will be a fine snack and you will not gain weight. However, there are other good reasons to eat not only peanuts but other nuts as well in moderation. The famous Nurses' Health Study study clearly shows that eating nuts was inversely associated with total and cause-specific mortality, independent of other predictors of death.[2] This was also seen in another study in the *New England Journal of Medicine*, which states in short that eating nuts prevents you from getting a variety of chronic diseases[3] including diabetes, a point also made in a nice study in *Diabetes Care*.[4] The lay literature is rife with articles on the beneficial effects of eating nuts, especially the fact that people who eat nuts seem to be skinnier. An excellent article on this topic is Jane Brody's *New York Times* blog post on snacking.[5]

Is it okay to eat vegetables?
Of course! The more you eat, the better. Just like fruits, vegetables are high in antioxidants. They will not stimulate the addiction center of the brain as the Addictocarbs do, but you still have to remember that even vegetable calories can sometimes add up, especially legumes. So, for instance, I would not eat two pounds of chickpeas.

What about coffee, alcohol, and tea?
Coffee is an addictive stimulant, and I would be remiss as a physician if I condoned it. That being said, let's face it, almost everyone drinks coffee. Many of my patients who are doctors also drink it. So if you are going to drink coffee, okay, but one patient came up with what I consider a stupendous idea and a guilty pleasure: She puts a spoon of Slimfast in it. It is sort of a play on Irish coffee, but with an Addictocarb Diet slant. It will be more filling, taste great, and hopefully put you off having a cupcake or croissant with that coffee.

I have similar feelings about alcohol. It is not good for you, and I do not drink; nevertheless, it is unlikely that I am going to convince anyone to stop drinking alcohol. The important thing here is how it relates to the Addictocarb Diet. The bottom line is that my patients have lost lots of weight while staying on the diet and continuing their alcohol consumption, so that is all I am concerned about. One patient pointed out an interesting fact to me. He was a big vodka drinker and mentioned that since vodka is usually made from potatoes, he switched to vodka that was made from berries. I had no idea such a thing existed, but I would love to hear from people who have other strategies like this on my website (http://www.Addictocarb.com).

In terms of tea, it is fine anytime, though I personally lean toward herbal teas like chamomile.

What about soda or diet soda?

I am always surprised when patients ask me this. Studies funded by the beverage industry keep coming out and claiming no link to obesity or any other malady. However, studies by just about everyone else suggest exactly the opposite. The long and the short of it is that soda is essentially liquid sugar, and because of that it has no place in an Addictocarb-free lifestyle. On the other hand, diet soda is not an Addictocarb.

So what of diet soda?[6] One study has shown that diet soda is associated with kidney decline.[7] Another study showed that drinking just one diet soda per day increases the risk of metabolic syndrome, which causes diabetes.[8] Yet another study has shown that the more diet soda a person drinks, the greater their risk of becoming overweight.[9] The thinking is that after eating diet foods, people are more likely to overeat because the body is being fooled into thinking it is eating sugar, and you just crave more. There has also been some discussion of the fact that mixing diet soda with alcohol causes the alcohol to enter the brain faster, and may result in a bigger hangover.[10] Furthermore, diet sodas also contain something many regular sodas don't—mold inhibitors, which may cause a host of problems such as hives and asthma.[11] Diet soda may be bad for your teeth, too.[12] On top of everything else, the cans and bottles may not be good for you,[13] even when they are BPA free.[14]

Can I use low-calorie sweeteners?

You will note in the recipe section of *The Addictocarb Diet* that I have a number of recipes that use sugar alternatives. I personally recommend whole-fruit puree as sweeteners, for which I also have recipes (see page 130). But alas, everything in life is about compromise; you cannot have everything you want. I think it would be best if you did not need to use any sweetener ever, but let's face it, that may not realistic. Note that even the non-calorie sweeteners have been shown in some studies to increase the risk of diabetes and make you feel compelled to eat more; therefore, I recommend you try not to use them.[15] There are, however, some things that simply require a little sweetness, and you may feel you need to use agave nectar, stevia, or the like. It's okay as long as you don't go overboard. I have not found that this leads to a cascade of addictive events.

Can I use bread crumbs?

Bread crumbs are made from bread. Bread is an Addictocarb, so you cannot have it. Here's an alternative: Patients have told me that when they needed to use bread crumbs—for instance, in meatballs—they have instead used the Wasa Crisp'n Light 7 Grain crackerbreads. They also use them for croutons in salads.

What juice can I drink?

You cannot drink any fruit juice, ever. Fruit juice is nothing more than liquid sugar—even if it's freshly squeezed. Vegetable juices, on the other hand, are great. You can make your own or buy them in the store. While I try to get organic when I can, I often just drink low-sodium V8 juice.

What about citrus fruits like grapefruits and oranges?

As a group, citrus fruits are not Addictocarbs. That is the good news. On the other hand, they are relatively high in calories and carbs. While the basic tenet of this diet is that calories and carbs do not matter, that is because if you stick to the diet you will not feel compelled to eat as many of them. Overall, however, calories do matter. You can eat bananas, but if you eat twenty-five in a day, the calories will add up. So the bottom line is, yes, you can have a grapefruit or an orange—just don't eat ten of them and certainly do not drink the juice.

Also consider why you are on this diet. If you are on this diet just to lose weight, grapefruits and oranges in moderation are fine. On the other hand, if you are a diabetic, you may have to consider them more carefully.

What if I am gluten free, lactose intolerant, or committed to a plant-based diet?

The Addictocarb Diet is a gluten-aware diet, and it's also sensitive to those who are lactose intolerant or eat a plant-based diet. For more information, see chapter nine: "Gluten Free, Lactose Free, Vegetarian, and More" (page 91).

What about organics?

I generally try to eat organic foods whenever possible, but I think that for certain things, organics are especially important, including milk, apples, pears, and peaches. I think you should *only* buy organic cow's milk (or soy or almond milk instead). Otherwise, you may be exposed to the many hormones and antibiotics in the milk. I also try to eat only organic fruit. This used to be quite difficult, but now all supermarkets have organic sections. Cascadian Farms frozen organic fruits are available almost everywhere, too. Two bags of Cascadian Farms frozen fruits is the perfect size for a Shake.

What if I prefer a plant-based diet?

Let's face it, being a vegan or a vegetarian presents significant but surmountable challenges in life. This is also true for the Addictocarb Diet. But it can be done. First, at its very base, the diet is about fruit. No problem there. Second, milk is important, but you can have almond or soy milk instead of cow's milk. You will also note that the recipe section has numerous vegetarian recipes.

SHAKE QUESTIONS

To read more about the Shake generally, see page 48.

How many Shakes can I drink?

As many as you want. The more the better.

How much fruit should I put into the Shake?

This is a moving target depending on the size of the blender that you use. I usually put in at least a pound of berries and at least a half a banana to about 3 ½ cups of milk. I believe more fruit is better, but you should do what tastes best to you.

Do I need to put a banana in the Shake?

No. You will lose more weight if you do not, just as you will lose more weight if you use water instead of milk or if you leave out the flavoring powder. The important thing is that the Shakes must be palatable in order for you to drink them. If it is palatable with half a banana, that's fine; if you need a whole banana to make it palatable, also fine. If you do not need any banana, then it's just as fine. I vary among using a whole banana, half, or none, but generally a half works for me. Patients have told me the same thing. I would not get too caught up in this, but just recall the discussion of the Japanese banana diet (page 57).

How long do I continue to use the Shakes?

I have been using the Shakes for ten years now. Patients tell me that they have worked the Shakes into the framework of their life. In general, the Shakes should be used exclusively for Step 1 of the diet and a lot in Step 2. In Step 3, use the Shakes over the years when going out to eat, if you fall off the wagon, or just as a healthy meal. After all, why not? It is a tasty, nutrition-packed alternative to eating fattening foods.

What to Eat and What to Avoid

STEP 1 (Duration: 3 days)

Eat:	Shakes, fruit (if craving/need to cheat), coffee
Don't eat:	Anything except for what is on the "Eat" list

STEP 2 (Duration: 2 weeks)

Eat:	sweet potatoes (boiled, baked, or fried), Wasa Crisp'n Light Crackerbreads (and anything made from them, including croutons), Dreamfields pasta, kasha, quinoa, wild rice, yogurt, cottage cheese, sour cream, coffee, tea, alcohol, meat, fish, chicken, turkey, tofu, beans, lentils, nuts of all kinds in moderation (especially almonds and peanuts), fruit (any type except figs and dates, including apples, pears, peaches, strawberries, raspberries, blackberries, blueberries, cantaloupe, watermelon, mangoes, grapefruits, lemons, limes, bananas, grapes, nectarines, pineapples, cherries), vegetables (carrots, cauliflower, broccoli, Brussels sprouts, beets, celery, onions, garlic, avocado, tomatoes, spinach, squash, mushrooms, eggplant, zucchini), vegetable juice, skim milk, nut milk (almond or cashew), soy milk, soy, unsweetened gum, Addictocarb-Free Pancakes (page 160), Cauliflower Pizza (page 137)
Don't eat:	• pasta (spaghetti, linguini, etc.), except for Dreamfields and quinoa pastas • flour (including cake, cookies, brownies, cupcakes, pancakes except for the recipe on page 160, breakfast cereals, waffles)

STEP 2 (Duration: 2 weeks), continued

Don't eat:
- rice (including rice cakes, rice wine, sushi, rice pasta, rice flour, fried rice, paella, rice crispies, rice noodles, rice cereal)

- sugar or sugary foods (including granola, table sugar, sweetened tea or coffee, sweetened alcoholic drinks like rum, ice cream)

- high fructose corn syrup (Check ingredients list on products to see if they contain this. Includes some ketchups; many breakfast cereals, syrups, salad dressings, and ice creams; some flavored yogurts; barbecue sauce; processed snacks; canned baked beans; canned fruit; some bottled applesauce; candy and candy bars; granola bars; and some health and nutrition bars.)

- fruit juice or anything that contains it

- candy (including milk chocolate, and any chocolate with less than 65 percent cacao)

- soda (diet or regular)

- potatoes (including French fries, baked potatoes, potato rolls, potato salad, home fries, mashed potatoes, potato chips, potato soup, potato skins, potato pancakes, potato gnocchi, and potato flakes

- bread, sandwiches (with bread), hamburger and hot dog rolls, olive bread, raisin bread, sourdough bread, rye bread, pumpernickel bread, corn bread, pizza, crackers of any kind except Wasa Crisp'n Light Crackerbreads, bagels, bread pudding, croutons, toast, tacos, quesadillas, burritos (except for the filling), chicken fried anything, French toast, and bread in store-bought meatballs and meatloaf

STEP 3 (Duration: Up to you, depending on how much weight you want to lose)

Eat:
There is no real difference between the foods you can and cannot eat between Steps 2 and 3. The main issue here is the decisions you have to make on how thin you want to be. You will become and stay as thin as you want based on the number of Addictocarbs you give up. For every Addictocarb you give up, you will be that much thinner. If you're trying to lose weight, continue to give up Addictocarbs until you reach your desired weight.

Some people, once they hit their target weight, will be fine just staying off bread and potatoes. Many people will also want to give up flour.

STEP 3 (Duration: Up to you, depending on how much weight you want to lose), continued

---

Eat: If you are a diabetic, you may need to give up most if not all Addictocarbs, but remember you can always have Addictocarb Alternatives for bread, rice, and potatoes and, if you must, Addictocarb Accommodations such as whole wheat pasta or brown rice.

Just bear in mind that every time you give up an Addictocarb it becomes that much easier to give up the next one.

The Addictocarb Diet Self-Assessment Tool (ADSAT)

The ADSAT was developed by two physicians, Kenneth Paul Rosenberg, M.D., a leading addiction specialist and author of the recently published medical textbook *Behavioral Addictions*; and Bruce Roseman, M.D., creator of the Addictocarb Diet. The point of the ADSAT is to help you determine if you are exhibiting addictive behaviors related to food, to identify those behaviors, and to be able to follow them over time to see how you are responding to the treatment regimen. The tool is meant not only to evaluate but to provoke a thought process about food addiction.

QUESTION	Never 0	Sometimes 1	Often 2	Always 3
Do you feel guilty about your eating or weight?				
Do you ever feel that you should stop eating but just feel powerless to stop?				
Have you ever thrown food away only to retrieve it later?				
Do you feel you are always going on and off a diet?				
Have you ever eaten a large and fully satisfying meal, only to catch the aroma of pizza, French fries, or freshly baked bread and feel the sudden urge to eat some, even though you know you are definitely not hungry?				
When you eat pasta, cake, bread, and/or other carbs, do you eat a portion or do you keep eating until you have eaten all there is?				
When you have cut down on certain foods, do you feel cranky and upset?				
Do you feel remorse when you eat too much?				
Do you find that you have a desire to eat certain foods, and when you try to cut down or stop eating them you feel greater desire for them?				
Do you know certain foods will cause you medical problems but still eat them anyway?				

QUESTION	Never 0	Sometimes 1	Often 2	Always 3
Have you been on diets over the years, and then just end up gaining the weight back?				
How often do you eat bread or potatoes at a given meal?				
How often in a given day do you sense that you are starving?				
Have you ever tried unsuccessfully to cut down on your food intake?				
Have you ever been annoyed by doctors, friends, or other people telling you to control your food intake?				
Do you find yourself eating not to satisfy hunger, but to satisfy emotional needs?				
When you see or smell a certain food, do you feel there is a compulsion to eat regardless of whether you are hungry or not?				

TOTALS: Add up the columns, write the totals in the boxes to the right and total them. Look at the explanation for your score below or go to http://www.Addictocarb.com to check your results.

Scoring:
30 or higher: You have a severe food addiction issue that *needs* to be addressed and you *need* the Addictocarb Diet.
20–30: You have food addiction issues that *should* be addressed, and you *should* be on the Addictocarb Diet.
10–20: You have some food addiction issues, but your problem is not severe and can probably be *easily* remedied by the Addictocarb Diet.
Less than 10: Probably no problem unless you have multiple 3s, but I have seen people even here benefit from the Addictocarb Diet.

The Addictocarb Diet Progress Tool

This tool is meant to help you evaluate your level of addiction and how you are progressing. You can go back to this tool at any time, and the responses will give you a reasonable idea of where you stand with your food addiction.

Make a list of the top foods that you crave. I have a basic list of foods that most people are addicted to, but everyone is different. To follow your addiction progress, you need to see for yourself if you are still craving certain foods. What I have observed with most people is that most of their cravings cease after Step 1. The problem after that is being exposed to situations where you break the diet, eat an Addictocarb, and the cravings return. You just have to restart the diet, and you can follow your progress on the chart. You will see your progress on the addiction. It is the premise of this diet that as long as your addictions are ceasing, you will continue to lose weight.

Day 0: Circle the food(s) you crave before starting the diet.	Day 3: Circle the foods you crave now.	Day 10: Circle the foods you crave now.	Day 20: Circle the foods you crave now.	Day 40: Circle the foods you crave now.
bread	bread	bread	bread	bread
pasta	pasta	pasta	pasta	pasta
potatoes	potatoes	potatoes	potatoes	potatoes
rice	rice	rice	rice	rice
flour	flour	flour	flour	flour
high fructose corn syrup	high fructose corn syrup	high fructose corn syrup	high fructose corn syrup	high fructose corn syrup
cake	cake	cake	cake	cake
cookies	cookies	cookies	cookies	cookies
juice	juice	juice	juice	juice
soda	soda	soda	soda	soda
chips	chips	chips	chips	chips
fries	fries	fries	fries	fries

Recipe Index

Index

Notes

Chapter 1

1 US Department of Agriculture, *The Agricultural Fact Book 2001–2002* (Reno, NV: The Delano Max Wealth Institute, LLC., 2011): http://www.usda.gov/documents/usda-factbook-2001-2002.pdf.

2 American Diabetes Association, "Statistics about Diabetes," June 10, 2014, last modified September 10, 2014, http://www.diabetes.org/diabetes-basics/statistics/.

Chapter 2

1 American Society of Addiction Medicine, "For the Public: Definition of Addiction," April 19, 2011, http://www.asam.org/for-the-public/definition-of-addiction.

2 Allison Aubrey, "Can You Be Addicted to Carbs? Scientists Are Checking That Out," *The Salt* (blog), NPR, June 26, 2013, http://www.npr.org/blogs/thesalt/2013/06/26/195292850/can-you-be-addicted-to-carbs-scientists-are-checking-that-out.

3 Ashley N. Gearhardt, Sonja Yokum, Patrick T. Orr, Eric Stice, William R. Corbin, and Kelly D. Brownell, "Neural Correlates of Food Addiction," *Archives of General Psychiatry* 68, no. 8 (2011): 808–816.

4 Belinda S. Lennerz et al., "Effects of Dietary Glycemic Index on Brain Regions Related to Reward and Craving in Men," *American Journal of Clinical Nutrition* 98, no. 3 (2013): 641–47, doi:10.3945/ajcn.113.064113.

5 Kenneth Paul Rosenberg and Laura Curtiss Feder, eds., *Behavioral Addictions: Criteria, Evidence, and Treatment* (San Diego, CA: Academic Press, 2014).

6 Food Addiction Institute, "DSM-V Acknowledges Food Addiction," August 18, 2013, http://foodaddictioninstitute.org/news-and-events/dsm-v-acknowledges-food-addiction/2013/08/.

7 Maia Szalavitz, "Heroin vs. Häagen-Dazs: What Food Addiction Looks Like in the Brain," *Time*, April 4, 2011, http://healthland. time.com/2011/04/04/heroin-vs-haagen-dazs-what-food -addiction-looks-like-in-the-brain/.

8 "Hooked: Why Bad Habits Are Hard to Break," *60 Minutes*, April 30, 2012, transcript and embedded video, 13:31, http://www .cbsnews.com/news/hooked-why-bad-habits-are-hard-to-break/.

9 "Dr. Nora Volkow, Director of the National Institute on Drug Abuse: 'Food Can Be as Addictive as Drugs,'" *Mental Health Treatment* (blog), accessed December 14, 2014, http://mentalhealth treatment.net/blog/is-food-addiction-real-nida-director-says- yes/.

10 Kelly D. Brownell, M. R. C. Greenwood, Eliot Stellar, and E. Eileen Shrager, "The Effects of Repeated Cycles of Weight Loss and Regain in Rats," *Physiology & Behavior* 38, no. 4 (1986): 459–64, http://www.sciencedirect.com/science/article /pii/0031938486904117?np=.

11 Wendy C. King et al., "Prevalence of Alcohol Use Disorders before and after Bariatric Surgery," *Journal of the American Medical Association* 307, no. 23 (2012): 2516–25.

Chapter 3

1 "Diet NOT Exercise Is the Key to Weight Loss, Claims Leading Personal Trainer," *The Mail Online*, August 23, 2013, http://www .dailymail.co.uk/health/article-2400962/Reluctant-gym-goers -rejoice-Diet-NOT-exercise-key-weight-loss-claims-leading -personal-trainer.html.

2 CB Ebbeling et al., "Effects of Dietary Composition on Energy Expenditure during Weight-Loss Maintenance," *Journal of the American Medical Association* 207, no. 24 (2012): 2627–34.

3 Sophie Egan, "Making the Case for Fruit," *Well* (blog), *New York Times*, July 31, 2013, http://well.blogs.nytimes.com/2013/07/31 /making-the-case-for-eating-fruit/.

4 "Why Is It Important to Eat Fruit?", ChooseMyPlate.gov, accessed December 14, 2014, http://www.choosemyplate.gov /food-groups/fruits-why.html.

Chapter 4

1 Emily J. Dhurandhar et al., "The Effectiveness of Breakfast Recommendations on Weight Loss: A Randomized Controlled Trial," *American Journal of Clinical Nutrition* 100, no. 2 (2014): 507–13.

2 Gretchen Reynolds, "Is Breakfast Overrated?", *Well* (blog), *New York Times*, August 21, 2014, http://well.blogs.nytimes .com/2014/08/21/is-breakfast-overrated/.

Chapter 5

1 Hong Wang, Guohua Cao, and Ronald L. Prior, "Total Anti-oxidant Capacity of Fruits," *Journal of Agricultural and Food Chemistry* 44, no. 3 (1996): 701–6; Guohoua Cao, Emin Sofic, and Ronald L. Prior, "Antioxidant Capacity of Tea and Common Vegetables," *Journal of Agricultural and Food Chemistry* 44, no. 11 (1996): 3426–43; Ronald L. Prior et al., "Antioxidant Capacity As Influenced by Total Phenolic and Anthocyanin Content, Maturity, and Variety of *Vaccinium* Species," *Journal of Agricultural and Food Chemistry* 46, no. 7 (1998): 2686–93.

2 M. A. Parelman et al., "Dietary Strawberry Powder Reduces Blood Glucose Concentrations in Obese and Lean C57BL/6 Mice, and Selectively Lowers Plasma C-reactive Protein in Lean Mice," *British Journal of Nutrition* 108, no. 10 (2012): 1789–99, doi:10.1017/S0007114512000037.

3 Gary D. Stoner et al., "Protection against Esophageal Cancer in Rodents with Lyophilized Berries: Potential Mechanisms," *Nutrition and Cancer* 54, no. 1 (2006): 33–46.

4 "Strawberries Stimulate Metabolism and Suppress Appetite," *Natural News*, June 25, 2010, http://www.naturalnews .com/029068_strawberries_metabolism.html.

5 S. M. Hannum, "Potential Impact of Strawberries on Human Health: A Review of the Science," *Critical Reviews in Food Science and Nutrition* 44, no. 1 (2004): 1–17.

6 Driscoll's, "Nutrition & Health: Strawberry Nutrition," accessed December 14, 2014, http://www.driscolls.com/nutrition-health /berry-nutrition-facts/strawberry-nutrition.

7 Mary Anne Durkin, "Strawberries Ease Inflammation," Arthritis Foundation, accessed December 14, 2014, http://www .arthritistoday.org/what-you-can-do/eating-well/arthritis-diet /strawberries-inflammation.php.

8 B. Burton-Freeman, A. Linares, D. Hyson, and T. Kappagoda, "Strawberry Modulates LDL Oxidation and Postprandial Lipemia in Response to High-Fat Meal in Overweight Hyperlipidemic Men and Women," *Journal of the American College of Nutrition* 29, no. 1 (2010): 46–54.

9   Cascadian Farm Organic, "Frozen Fruit" (product description), 2013, accessed December 14, 2014, http://www.cascadianfarm .com/products/frozen-fruit.

10 Cascadian Farm Organic, "Premium Organic Red Raspberries" (product description), 2013, accessed December 14, 2014, http://www.cascadianfarm.com/products/product_detail .aspx?cat=9&upc=0-21908-53001-7.

11 Louise Atkinson, "Eat Carbs, Lose Weight: How Carbohydrates Can Help You Eat Less AND Burn More Calories," *Daily Mail* (online), June 6, 2011, http://www.dailymail.co.uk/femail/article -1394616/Diet-carbohydrates-help-lose-weight.html.

12 J. A. Gilbert et al., "Milk Supplementation Facilitates Appetite Control in Obese Women during Weight Loss: A Randomised, Single-Blind, Placebo-Controlled Trial," *British Journal of Nutrition* 105, no. 1 (2011): 133–43.

13 A. R. Josse, S. A. Atkinson, M. A. Tarnopolsky, and S. M. Phillips, "Increased Consumption of Dairy Foods and Protein during Diet- and Exercise-Induced Weight Loss Promotes Fat Mass Loss and Lean Mass Gain in Overweight and Obese Premenopausal Women," *Journal of Nutrition* 141, no. 9 (2011): 1626–34.

14 G. Wagner, S. Kindrick, S. Hertzler, and R. A. DiSilvestro, "Effects of Various Forms of Calcium on Body Weight and Bone Turnover Markers in Women Participating in a Weight Loss Program," *Journal of the American College of Nutrition* 26, no. 5 (2007): 456–61.

Chapter 6

1   Dreamfields Foods, "Healthy Pasta That Tastes Like Traditional Pasta!" (product page), 2014, accessed December 14, 2014, http:// www.dreamfieldsfoods.com/faq-search.php#!prettyPhoto/1/.

2   Pectin, xanthan gum, inulin, wheat gluten, and potassium chloride.

Chapter 7

1   2013 International Year of Quinoa Secretariat, Food and Agricultural Organization of the United Nations, "Quinoa 2013 International Year," accessed December 14, 2014, http://www .fao.org/quinoa-2013/en/.

2   Jolinda Hackett, "What Is Quinoa? Definition of Quinoa and Quinoa Recipes," *About Food*, accessed December 14, 2014, http://

vegetarian.about.com/od/glossary/g/whatisquinoa.htm; Laura Dolson, "Carbs in Quinoa," *About Health,* accessed December 14, 2014, http://lowcarbdiets.about.com/od/CarbsInGrains/a/Carbs-In-Quinoa.htm.

Chapter 9

1 National Institute of Diabetes and Digestive and Kidney Diseases, "Lactose Intolerance: Who Is More Likely to Have Lactose Intolerance?", last modified June 4, 2014, http://digestive.niddk.nih.gov/ddiseases/pubs/lactoseintolerance/#who.

2 Susan S. Lang, "Lactose Intolerance Seems Linked to Ancestral Struggles with Harsh Climate and Cattle Diseases, Cornell Study Finds," *Cornell Chronicle,* June 1, 2005, http://www.news.cornell.edu/stories/2005/06/lactose-intolerance-linked-ancestral-struggles-climate-diseases.

3 Michael Kerr, "Is It Crohn's Disease or Lactose Intolerance?", *Healthline,* March 7, 2012, http://www.healthline.com/health/crohns-disease/lactose-intolerance.

Chapter 11

1 *Dictionary.com,* s.v. "Snack," accessed December 14, 2014, http://dictionary.reference.com/browse/snack?s=t.

2 L. B. Sørensen and A. Astrup, "Eating Dark and Milk Chocolate: A Randomized Crossover Study of Effects on Appetite and Energy intake," *Nutrition and Diabetes* 1 (2011, December 5): e21, doi:10.1038/nutd.2011.17.

3 Dirk Taubert, Reinhard Berkels, Renate Roesen, and Wolfgang Klaus, "Chocolate and Blood Pressure in Elderly Individuals with Isolated Systolic Hypertension," *Journal of the American Medical Association* 290, no. 8 (2003): 1029–30, http://jama.jamanetwork.com/article.aspx?doi=10.1001/jama.290.8.1029.

4 K. W. Lee, Y. J. Kim, H. J. Lee, and C. Y. Lee, "Cocoa Has More Phenolic Phytochemicals and a Higher Antioxidant Capacity Than Teas and Red Wine," *Journal of Agricultural and Food Chemicals* 51, no. 25 (2003): 7292–95.

Chapter 12

1 Ioannis Protopsaltis et al., "Linking Pre-Diabetes with Benign Prostate Hyperplasia. IGFBP-3: A Conductor of Benign Prostate Hyperplasia Development Orchestra?", *PLoS One* 8, no. 12 (2013): e81411. doi:10.1371/journal.pone.0081411.

2   E. Giovannucci et al., "Obesity and Benign Prostatic Hyper-
    plasia," *American Journal of Epidemiology* 140, no. 11 (1994):
    989–1002; A. R. Kristal et al., "Race/Ethnicity, Obesity, Health
    Related Behaviors and the Risk of Symptomatic Benign Pros-
    tatic Hyperplasia: Results from the Prostate Cancer Prevention
    Trial," *Journal of Urology* 177, no. 4 (2007): 1395–1400.
3   Stephen J. Freedland, "Obesity and Prostate Cancer: A Growing
    Problem," *Clinical Cancer Research* 11 (October 1, 2005): 6763.
4   National Cancer Institute, "Obesity and Cancer Risk," reviewed
    January 3, 2012, http://www.cancer.gov/cancertopics/factsheet
    /Risk/obesity.

Chapter 13
1   Diabetes Prevention Program Research Group, "Reduction in
    the Incidence of Type 2 Diabetes with Lifestyle Intervention or
    Metformin," *New England Journal of Medicine* 346 (2002): 346,
    393–403, doi:10.1056/NEJMoa012512.
2   American Diabetes Association, "Statistics about Diabetes,"
    last modified September 10, 2014, http://www.diabetes.org
    /diabetes-basics/diabetes-statistics/.
3   George Alberti et al., "Type 2 Diabetes in the Young: The Evolv-
    ing Epidemic," *Diabetes Care* 27, no. 7 (2004): 1798–1811.
4   Dana Dabelea et al., "Prevalence of Type 1 and Type 2 Diabetes
    among Children and Adolescents from 2001 to 2009," *Journal
    of the American Medical Association* 311, no. 17 (2014): 1778–86,
    doi:10.1001/jama.2014.3201.
5   ABSI calculator, http://www-ce.ccny.cuny.edu/nir/sw/absi
    -calculator.html.
6   American Diabetes Association, "Diagnosing Diabetes and
    Learning about Prediabetes," last modified September 22, 2014,
    http://www.diabetes.org/diabetes-basics/diagnosis/.

Chapter 18
1   Alam Khan et al., "Cinnamon Improves Glucose and Lipids of
    People with Type 2 Diabetes," *Diabetes Care* 26, no. 12 (2003):
    3215–18.
2   A. M. Hutchins et al., "Daily Flaxseed Consumption Improves
    Glycemic Control in Obese Men and Women with Pre-diabetes:
    A Randomized Study," *Nutrition Research* 33, no. 5 (2013): 367–
    75, doi:10.1016/j.nutres.2013.02.012.

Appendix A

1 J. A. Linde et al., "Self-Weighing in Weight Gain Prevention and Weight Loss Trials," *Annals of Behavioral Medicine* 30, no. 3 (2005): 210–16.

2 Ying Bao et al., "Association of Nut Consumption with Total and Cause-Specific Mortality," *New England Journal of Medicine* 369, no. 21 (2013): 2001–11.

3 Ibid.

4 D. J. Jenkins et al., "Nuts as a Replacement for Carbohydrates in the Diabetic Diet," *Diabetes Care* 34, no, 8 (2011): 1706–11, doi:10.2337/dc11-0338.

5 Jane Brody, "Snacking Your Way to Better Health," *Well* (blog), *New York Times*, December 9, 2013, http://well.blogs.nytimes.com/2013/12/09/snacking-your-way-to-better-health/.

6 S. D. Stellman and L. Garfinkel, "Artificial Sweetener Use and One-Year Weight Change among Women," *Preventive Medicine* 15 (1986): 195–202.

7 J. Lin and G. C. Curhan, "Associations of Sugar and Artificially Sweetened Soda with Albuminuria and Kidney Function Decline in Women," *Clinical Journal of the American Society of Nephrology* 6, no. 1 (2011): 160–66.

8 Jennifer A. Nettleton et al., "Diet Soda Intake and Risk of Incident Metabolic Syndrome and Type 2 Diabetes in the Multi-Ethnic Study of Atherosclerosis," *Diabetes Care* 32, no. 4 (2009): 688–94.

9 Qing Yang, "Gain Weight by 'Going Diet?' Artificial Sweeteners and the Neurobiology of Sugar Cravings," *Yale Journal of Biology and Medicine* 83, no. 2 (2010): 101–8.

10 Mandy Oaklander, "7 Side Effects of Drinking Diet Soda," *Yahoo! Canada Shine*, September 17, 2012, https://ca.shine.yahoo.com/7-side-effects-of-drinking-diet-soda.html.

11 Ibid.

12 Ibid.

13 Ibid.

14 Sarah Toland, "Why BPA-Free Plastic Isn't Necessarily Safe," *Men's Journal*, accessed December 14, 2014, http://www.mensjournal.com/health-fitness/health/why-bpa-free-plastic-isnt-necessarily-safe-20140611.

15 Yang, "Gain Weight by 'Going Diet?'"

About the Author

Dr. Bruce Roseman has been a family doctor in private practice in Manhattan for thirty years and is affiliated with Mount Sinai Hospital, where he holds joint appointments in the departments of Family Medicine and Ob/Gyn. He has served as medical editor for several food/health-related books and magazines, including *The Olive Oil Cookbook*, *The Low Cholesterol Oat Cure*, Whittle's *The Health Report*, and *Big Bird Goes to the Doctor* (Sesame Street), and as a medical columnist for *Woman's World*. He has appeared on numerous television and radio programs as a medical expert, including *Live Wire* (PBS), *The Human Condition* (NPR), *Good Day New York*, *The Queen Latifah Show*, and *The Joan Lunden Show*, and has been featured in magazines such as *Guideposts* and *Parent*. He is the author of *A Kid Just Like Me* (Penguin/Putnam, 2001), which details a popular method he invented, while working with his son, to teach children with learning disabilities to read. He lives happily in New York City with his wife of over a quarter century, Ellen, and is proud to be the father of two fine young men, Joshua and Aaron.